DASH DIET MEAL PREP

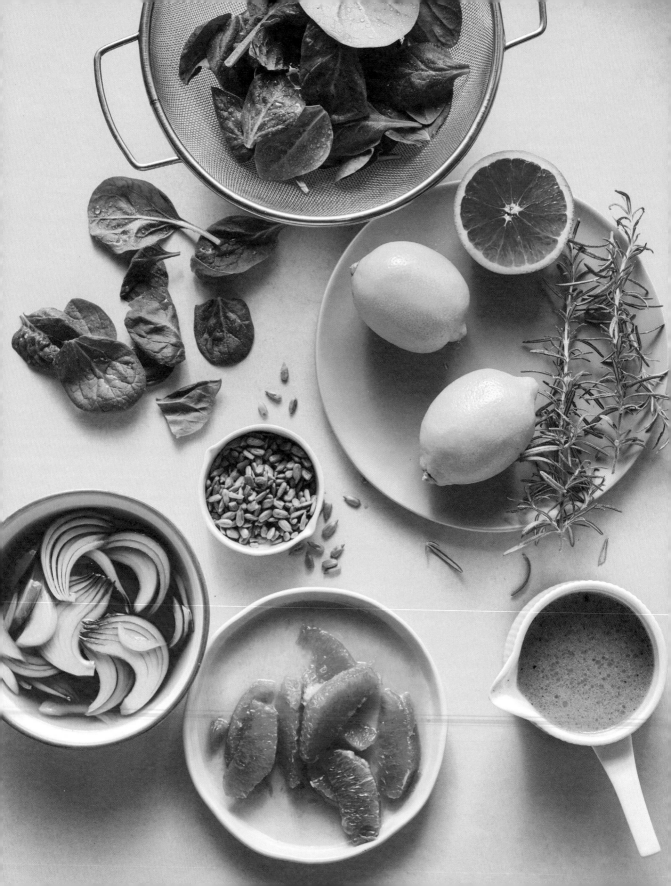

DASH DIET MEAL PREP

100 Healthy Recipes and 6 Weekly Plans

MARIA-PAULA CARRILLO, MS, RDN, LD
&
KATIE MCKEE, MCN, RDN, LD

Photography by Antonis Achilleos

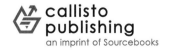

callisto
publishing
an imprint of Sourcebooks

Published by Callisto Publishing LLC C/O Sourcebooks LLC
P.O. Box 4410, Naperville, Illinois 60567-4410
(630) 961-3900
callistopublishing.com

Printed and bound in China
OGP 2

MARIA-PAULA:

To my husband, Chris, my biggest cheerleader and support; my mom, Maria-Paula, who prepares all her dishes with so much love and flavor; and my daughters, Victoria and Sophia, who tried every recipe and will always be my inspiration for good food and healthy bodies.

───────

KATIE:

To my mom, Kiki, who brings everyone to her table; my aunts, Sue and Julie, who built communities with food; my grandmother Trini, who always had something for us to try; and Sean and Milo, who tasted these recipes and washed the dishes.

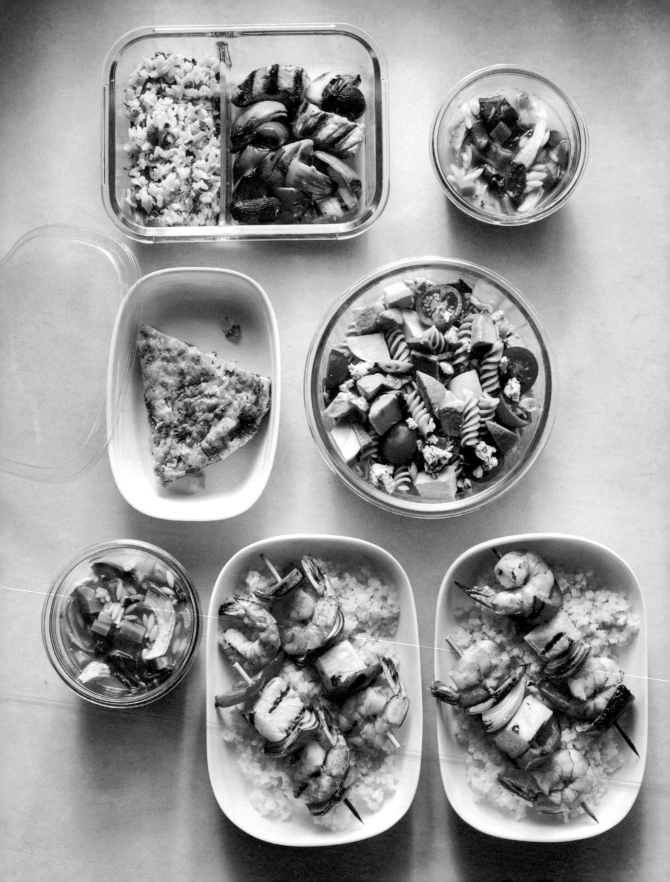

CONTENTS

INTRODUCTION

In a hectic world, eating healthy can be challenging. With careers, commitments—and in some cases, kids—getting to the grocery store, cooking, and connecting at the dinner table may be close to impossible. As registered dietitian nutritionists, we know the many benefits of eating healthier. As moms, we also know the struggle of getting it all done.

―――――

We may not be able to solve all your food problems, but we can help you streamline your week, providing healthy recipes, shopping lists, step-by-step instructions, and a lot of encouragement along the way. As dietitians, we know the science behind the DASH diet and how it can truly benefit your health. We also know that simplifying your diet with meal prep can be integral to creating new habits, and we hope we can help you develop a healthier diet that will stick and is also good for everyone in your household.

One of the best things about the DASH diet is that it is versatile. It uses all five food groups and includes many foods that you already enjoy. It's a great road map for healthier eating, and *you* get to decide where to go. As dietitians, we want to help you embrace flavors and foods you like with a healthier spin. It's beneficial to personalize the DASH diet in ways that make sense for you. Eating for better health inspires both of us in different ways.

Katie is a skeptic and so, when it comes to a scientific claim, always wants to see the study. She sets goals, works hard, and pushes her friends and family to do the same. Maria-Paula is an expert on food allergies, gastrointestinal disorders, and pediatric nutrition. In her practice, she translates the science of healthy eating into strategies that work for families. Katie strives for simplicity in her kitchen, looking toward the California coast for her inspiration. She also tries to introduce her preschooler, Milo, to new foods, hoping he'll embrace a love for nutrition and cooking. So far, so good. Maria-Paula truly believes all foods can be a part of a healthy diet when we create balance in our meals and snacks. As a mother of two daughters, Victoria and Sophia, she strives to leave behind the diet mentality, sharing and embracing the reality that food is nourishment, strength, and vitality.

With the DASH diet, Katie believes that the science will keep you going on those days when you simply don't want to do any more prep. Maria-Paula knows that flavor is the main reason anyone chooses a meal, and she's sure that building confidence in the kitchen and being adaptable with recipes will be your keys to success. In this book, you'll find evidence of two quite different dietitians with two different approaches who decided to collaborate—a recipe for the perfect balance of nutrition and taste. We may be different but we have a shared vision: We both believe that food is central to our lives as dietitians, as moms, as daughters, and as friends. We view food as medicine and have seen the positive change good nutrition can have for families.

At the end of the day, both of us strive to spend time with our families around the table—whether it be around the kitchen island after a long evening of sport practices, laughing while sharing a meal with friends, or a Sunday night dinner reflecting on the week ahead. We hope we can inspire you to bring good food to your table and to share it with the ones you love.

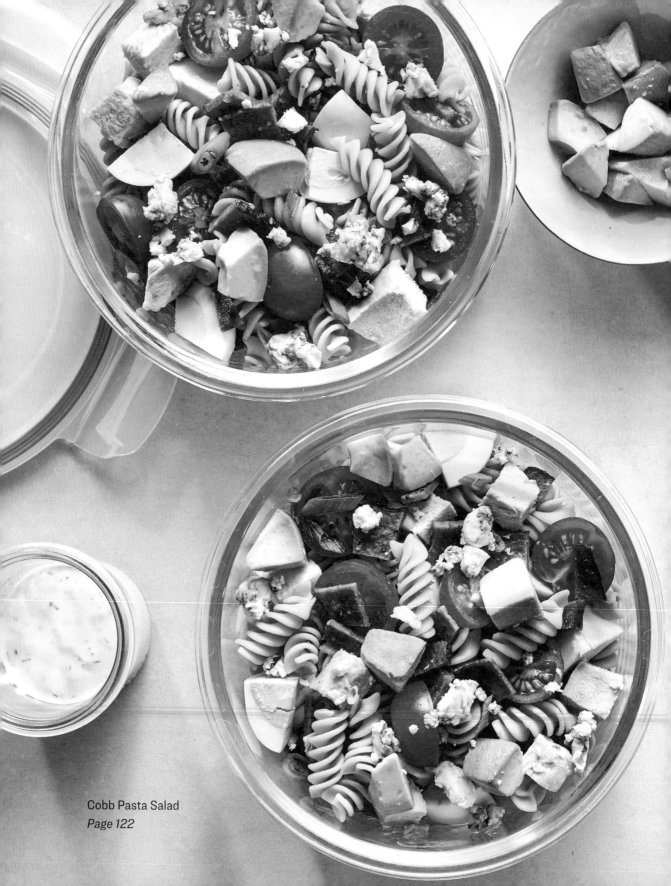

Cobb Pasta Salad
Page 122

PART ONE

DASH MADE EASY

People often jump into a new diet with fear and hesitation. With DASH, there's no reason to be fearful. Most of the diet will sound familiar. It may be prescribed for those with high blood pressure, but it benefits just about everyone. The diet doesn't stray far from recommendations made in current federal nutrition guidelines. And combining the DASH diet with meal prep allows you even greater control over what you eat and your grocery budget. In this first part, we'll explain the extensive science behind DASH and give you the tools and ingredients needed for long-term success.

Veggie Frittata
Page 44

CHAPTER 1

Ready to DASH

Simply put, DASH is a flexible diet that involves seeking specific foods encompassing all five food groups—fruits, vegetables, dairy, grains, and proteins. DASH is whole-food focused because you get so much more with whole foods versus supplements. When you combine certain foods, nutrients are enhanced. For instance, fruits rich in vitamin C help you absorb iron from your meats or leafy greens. And when you eat yogurt and whole grains together, the probiotics in the yogurt work with the prebiotics in the whole grains to provide more nutrients. Both help build beneficial bacteria in your gut.

In this chapter, we'll dive into the science behind DASH to understand why doctors and dietitians have recommended it for years. We'll put the principles into practice by identifying better-for-you foods, better-for-you seasonings, and better-for-you cooking techniques. Finally, we'll focus on which foods you should choose and which to avoid as you build your plate. With a better understanding of why you should adopt the DASH diet and how easy it can be, you'll be dashing toward a new lifestyle of healthy foods and seeing health benefits in no time.

WHAT IS DASH?

DASH stands for the **D**ietary **A**pproaches to **S**top **H**ypertension. It's an eating pattern developed to prevent and treat high blood pressure and promote heart health. According to the Centers for Disease Control and Prevention, one in three American adults (75 million) have high blood pressure, and another one in three American adults have higher than normal blood pressure. High blood pressure is known as the silent killer; many people do not know they have it since it has no signs or symptoms. When left untreated, high blood pressure damages the circulatory system and can lead to kidney damage, heart attack, heart failure, and stroke. Reducing risk factors, making lifestyle changes, and overhauling how you eat can lower blood pressure. DASH is a perfect place to start.

DASH has more than 20 years of research behind it. Developed by the National Heart, Lung, and Blood Institute, DASH has been studied in many different populations, including those underrepresented in traditional research: African Americans and women. It places a focus on reducing sodium while increasing potassium, magnesium, calcium, fiber, and protein. It recommends:

- Eating fruits, vegetables, whole grains, and low-fat or nonfat dairy products, as well as legumes, nuts, lean poultry, and fish
- Limiting high-sodium foods, sweets, sugary beverages, and some red meats

One of the best features of the DASH diet is that the foods recommended are likely foods you already eat. They also closely reflect the federal Dietary Guidelines for Americans, better known as MyPlate. Another perk about DASH is that it can work quite quickly—some see their blood pressure drop by a few points within two weeks, and over time, drop to a level that makes a significant difference in other health risk factors.

DASH HEALTH BENEFITS

The DASH diet is a favorite of doctors, dietitians, and allied health professionals because it's well researched, easy to follow, effective, and sustainable. DASH isn't a fad diet. It's a healthier eating plan that will benefit you now and in the future. There are many reasons that DASH ranks as one of the best overall diets in *U.S. News & World Report* year after year. Here are a few of the benefits you might experience.

Lower blood pressure. DASH provides generous amounts of key nutrients that play a part in lowering blood pressure, including potassium, magnesium, calcium, protein, and fiber. Decades of research have shown that following DASH can lead to a reduction in blood pressure for both healthy and hypertensive adults. Follow-up studies have shown greater reductions in blood pressure with reduced sodium intake.

Reduced cancer risk. Recent findings in the *Journal of Research in Medical Sciences* found that people following DASH had a lower risk of some cancers, including colorectal and breast cancer.

Reduced diabetes risk. A recent study in *Diabetes Spectrum* highlighted DASH benefits, including promoting blood pressure control, weight loss, and improved insulin resistance and cholesterol levels.

Reduced osteoporosis risk. The blood pressure–reducing minerals favored by DASH— calcium and potassium—are also bone healthy. Add a little vitamin D and protein, both found in DASH-friendly recipes, and you have a great foundation for bone health.

Reduced risk of heart disease. DASH plays a protective role against cardiovascular diseases, coronary heart disease, stroke, and heart failure. It also works to lower cholesterol.

Weight loss. Although it wasn't originally designed for weight loss, DASH provides low-calorie, high-fiber, high-protein foods that help alleviate hunger and aid satiety. It also cuts out a lot of high-fat and high-sugar foods, which can help you shed unwanted pounds.

DASH DIET GUIDELINES

The DASH diet is rich in fruits, vegetables, whole grains, lean protein, and low-fat or nonfat dairy. You'll focus on selecting whole foods from all five food groups, providing you the nutrients you need to lose weight and lower blood pressure naturally. Research also shows great benefit to sodium restriction. In DASH diet trials, the more that sodium was restricted, the greater the drop in blood pressure for the individual. We're not asking you to limit all sodium or cut out everything you enjoy. Focusing on a few simple solutions should help you meet your health goals. Let's look at a few best practices for your meals.

Add nuts, seeds, and legumes. These are good sources of magnesium, potassium, and protein. They're also full of fiber, phytochemicals, and healthy fats, including monounsaturated fat and omega-3 fatty acids.

Choose lean proteins. Lean cuts of meat, poultry, and fish provide a range of nutrients, including B vitamins, vitamin E, iron, zinc, and magnesium. Animal protein is also a high-quality, complete protein, meaning it contains all the essential amino acids. Limit choices that are high in saturated fat to keep your cholesterol levels healthy.

Consider your calories when it comes to dairy.
Dairy foods are a great source of three nutrients doctors recommend for healthy blood pressure: calcium, potassium, and magnesium. They're also packed with high-quality protein. A study in the *American Journal of Clinical Nutrition* found that when whole-fat dairy foods were incorporated into the DASH diet, participants maintained the heart-healthy benefits. Switching to low-fat or nonfat dairy may only benefit you when it comes to counting calories.

Eat more fruits and vegetables. A generous amount of fruits and vegetables each day provides essential nutrients, including potassium, fiber, folate, beta-carotene (vitamin A), and vitamin C. Plant foods also provide phytochemicals and antioxidants—compounds that protect our bodies, boost our immunity, and reduce risk of chronic disease.

Limit sodium intake. Many people think salt and sodium are interchangeable, but that's not quite true. Sodium is a mineral and is one of the components in salt; the other is chloride. DASH works best if you work to reduce your intake to no more than 1 teaspoon of salt a day (2,300 milligrams sodium). For some people, it is less than ¾ teaspoon of salt (1,500 milligrams sodium). If you aren't sure which sodium level is right for you, talk to your doctor.

Limit sugar and alcohol. An easy place to cut calories is added sugars and alcohol. Limit your sweets to fewer than five servings each week. Alcohol can also raise blood pressure. The Dietary Guidelines for Americans recommend that men limit alcohol to no more than two drinks a day, and women to one or less.

SNEAKY SODIUM

Sodium occurs naturally in some foods, such as milk, celery, and beets. But more than 75 percent of our sodium intake comes from preservatives in packaged foods at the grocery store and ordered at restaurants. Only about 11 percent comes from your saltshaker at home, according to the American Heart Association (AHA). A few foods that rank particularly high are known as the AHA's Salty Six:

- Breads and rolls
- Burritos and tacos
- Cold cuts and cured meats
- Pizza
- Sandwiches
- Soup

Aiming for a no-salt-added option is a good choice at the grocery store. Compare products using the nutrition facts label as a tool to manage sodium intake. And don't forget to check the serving size to make the most accurate comparison. Keep in mind that sodium isn't the only sneaky ingredient. Watch the nutrition facts label for sugar, too. It acts as a natural preservative and is found in many processed foods.

WHAT TO EAT (AND NOT EAT) ON THE DASH DIET

FOOD GROUP / ENJOY FREELY	EAT IN MODERATION (limited to ≤1 serving)	AVOID OR LIMIT
DAIRY Nonfat and 1%-fat milk, low-fat and nonfat cheese, low-fat and nonfat yogurt, low-fat and nonfat cottage cheese, low-fat and nonfat ricotta cheese, nonfat cream cheese, nonfat sour cream	2%-fat milk (8 ounces), low-fat cream cheese (1 tablespoon), low-fat sour cream (1 tablespoon)	Whole milk, full-fat cheese, regular sour cream, regular cream cheese, full-fat yogurt (if counting calories; see page 6 for more)
FRUITS Citrus, berries, bananas, grapes, melons, pineapples, mangos, peaches, apricots, apples, pears, plums, kiwis	Avocado (½), dried fruit (¼ cup)	None
GRAINS Whole wheat and whole-grain breads, whole-grain breakfast cereals, wheat germ, brown rice, bulgur, whole wheat couscous, quinoa, oatmeal	White bread (1 slice), white pasta (½ cup cooked), white rice (½ cup cooked)	Sugar-filled breakfast cereals, donuts, pastries, cakes, cookies, pies
FATS AND OILS Canola oil, olive oil, vegetable oil	Butter (1 teaspoon), mayonnaise (1 tablespoon), salad dressing (1 tablespoon)	Coconut oil, palm oil, lard, solid margarine
PROTEINS Lean poultry, fish, eggs, beans, legumes, tofu	Nuts and seeds (⅓ cup of nuts, 2 tablespoons of seeds, 2 tablespoons of nut butter), red meat (6 ounces or fewer)	Bacon, sausage, hot dogs, luncheon meats, and smoked, cured, or pickled foods
VEGETABLES Tomatoes, carrots, summer squash, broccoli, leafy greens, mushrooms, green beans, cabbage, cauliflower, asparagus, Brussels sprouts, onions	Winter squash (½ cup), corn (½ cup), green peas (⅔ cup)	None

Seek seafood. Seafood provides healthy omega-3 fatty acids. Eating about 8 ounces per week of a variety of seafood contributes to the prevention of heart disease by reducing risk factors, including high triglycerides, blood clot formation, and inflammation.

Swap out refined grains for whole grains. Whole-grain foods provide fiber, energy-producing B vitamins, and iron. They also aid in healthy digestion, weight management, and reducing the risk of heart disease.

Swap out saturated fats for healthy fats. Seek out polyunsaturated (PUFA) or monounsaturated (MUFA) fats for their essential fatty acids and high amounts of vitamin E. These fats—found in fish, plants, and nuts—do not raise LDL cholesterol. Fats contain 100 to 120 calories per serving (for example, 1 tablespoon of olive oil), so use sparingly to avoid excess calories.

CHOOSING THE RIGHT PORTION SIZES

Calorie needs vary based on age, sex, and level of activity. For adults, calorie needs can range from 1,600 to 3,000 calories per day. On a 2,000-calorie-a-day diet, you can estimate portion sizes using your hand:

- A fingertip represents a teaspoon of fats or oils.
- A fist is the size of a vegetable, fruit, milk, or yogurt serving.
- A flat full hand is the length of a slice of bread or a serving of fish.
- A handful is the right amount for rice, noodles, or oatmeal.
- A palm is the size of a serving of poultry or meat.
- A pointer finger is the size of a serving of string cheese.
- A thumb represents a tablespoon of a condiment or nut butter.

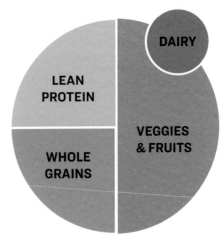

An easy way to put DASH diet principles into practice is to simply make a plate. Fill half your plate with fruits and vegetables, a quarter with whole grains, and a quarter with lean protein, and place a serving of dairy on the side. Add some nuts, beans, and seeds, and you're set. As we dive into our meal prep plan, we'll focus on adding delicious flavor through herbs, spices, and cooking techniques.

GO-TO DASH SWAPS

An easy way to eat closer to the DASH diet is to overhaul your ingredients. Finding the right fit will help you meet your goals without sacrificing great taste. Here are our top 10 to replace.

- **Butter.** Olive oil offers heart-healthy benefits and versatility. It works best with savory recipes, but can be used in some sweet recipes, too.

- **Cereal.** Oatmeal is a low-sugar, fiber-rich alternative.

- **High-fat cheese.** Hard, aged cheeses deliver a lot of flavor. Replace milder cheeses, such as mozzarella, provolone, or Cheddar with Gouda, Parmesan, or Romano, and save some calories, salt, and saturated fat.

- **Red meat.** Variety is the spice of life (and of the DASH diet). Every week, replace a few servings of red meat with heart-healthy DASH all-stars—fish, nuts, and beans—to maximize your health.

- **Salad dressing.** A simple dressing of olive oil, lemon juice, and herbes de Provence (a savory mix of marjoram, rosemary, thyme, oregano, and lavender) acts as a healthy and affordable replacement to a high-sodium dressing.

- **Salt.** Many different herbs and spices can fulfill the role salt plays—reducing bitterness and enhancing sweetness:

    > Basil pairs well with tomatoes, cheese, and vegetables. It also makes a great pesto sauce.

    > Cilantro works well with many chicken, seafood, beef, and grain-based dishes. Think about adding it to a quinoa bowl with avocado or to a pork dish with brown rice.

    > Dill is great paired with fish. Consider topping tilapia or cod with it. It's also great in a creamy salad dressing made with Greek yogurt and a little lemon juice.

- **Sour cream.** Greek yogurt offers more protein and less fat. An additional benefit is that you can use the same amount in your recipes (1:1 ratio).

- **Sugar.** Cinnamon's slightly sweet taste makes it a great substitute for sugar. Combine it with Greek yogurt for the perfect topping to seasonal fresh fruit.

- **Sugary drinks.** Sports drinks, sodas, and sweet teas all provide empty calories. Focus on fruit-infused waters, sparkling waters, unsweetened teas, and kombucha instead.

- **White bread.** White bread is made with refined flour, which has lost many of its nutrients during processing. Seek out whole-grain breads and use whole wheat flour if making home-made bread (or pancakes). Also, incorporate other whole grains into your diet, such as brown rice and ancient grains like quinoa, for better digestion and improved heart health.

SIMPLE HERB SUBSTITUTES

Fresh herbs can be cumbersome. On days you want to ditch the work or swap something out of your pantry, we have you covered. Make this herb and garlic conversion chart your go-to for the perfect substitute.

HERB	FRESH	DRIED	FREEZE-DRIED	PASTE*
Basil	1 tablespoon	1 teaspoon	1 tablespoon	2 teaspoons
Cilantro	1 tablespoon	1 teaspoon	1 tablespoon	1 tablespoon
Dill	1 tablespoon	1 teaspoon	1 tablespoon	1 tablespoon
Garlic	1½ teaspoons minced (1 large clove)	½ teaspoon powder	1½ teaspoons	1½ teaspoons
Oregano	1 tablespoon	1 teaspoon	1 tablespoon	1 tablespoon
Parsley	2 teaspoons	1 teaspoon	2 teaspoons	2 teaspoons
Rosemary	1 tablespoon	1 tablespoon	1 tablespoon	1 tablespoon
Sage	2 teaspoons	1 teaspoon	2 teaspoons	2 teaspoons
Thyme	1 tablespoon	1 teaspoon (¾ teaspoon ground)	1 tablespoon	1 tablespoon

Some of these pastes won't be available at the grocery store, so you can blend them at home. They will keep for up to 2 weeks in the refrigerator but can also be frozen in ice cubes for later use. For the rosemary, sage, and thyme: Blend ½ cup of fresh herbs with 2½ tablespoons of extra-virgin olive oil.

Turkey Meatballs with Whole Wheat Penne in
Simple Tomato Sauce
Page 60

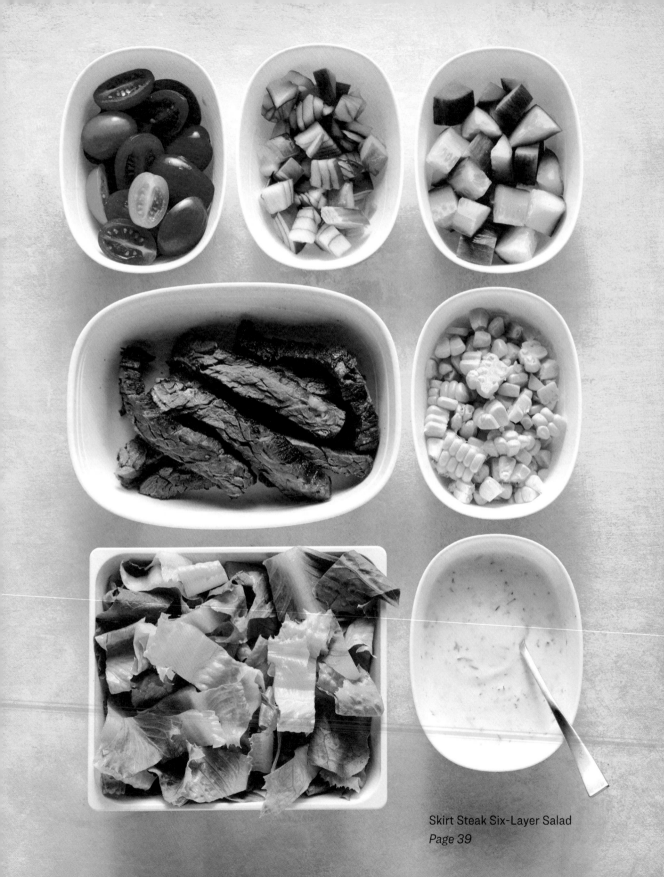

Skirt Steak Six-Layer Salad
Page 39

CHAPTER 2

What Meal Prep Is (and Why It Works Well with DASH)

Meal prepping may be your secret weapon for putting DASH into practice. It saves time, reduces waste, and keeps you accountable to your health and wellness goals. Forecasting your menu, getting the ingredients together, and prepping for a full week of meals that you can take on the go eliminates the guesswork of what to eat when you are tired and overwhelmed.

If you're just getting started with meal prepping, you might be feeling a little anxious. But don't worry, we're here to guide you. We will show you, step-by-step, how to prepare and streamline your meals so you can stay on track with your DASH diet plan.

WHY PREP?

When you start meal prepping, you may be pleasantly surprised by all the benefits it brings. Meal prepping:

Saves time. Using one day to plan and prepare your meals decreases the time you spend in the kitchen the rest of the week. That also means less time shopping, cooking, and cleaning, which gives you more time to spend on things you love.

Reduces waste. When you plan and prep your meals ahead of time, you can include recipes that feature the same ingredients. This will decrease the amount of food left unused (and possibly to spoil) in your refrigerator. Currently, Americans waste one-third of the food they buy each year. Meal prepping could be the start of a sustainable practice for you and the environment.

Helps you stick to your diet plan. Meal prepping allows you to choose foods and flavors that meet your cravings and nutrition goals. Meals that have been frozen can help you fill the gap when the unexpected happens.

Aids in portion control. Following DASH portion principles (see Choosing the Right Portion Sizes, page 8) and storing your food in individual containers makes it easy to get just what you need, and not too much. It also helps you be mindful during your meals—to savor your food rather than devour it out of hunger.

Improves your cooking skills. It goes without saying, but spending time preparing a variety of dishes each week will exponentially increase your confidence in the kitchen.

Saves money. Another benefit of reducing waste, planning, and making fewer last-minute grocery runs is that it saves you money.

MEAL PREP PRINCIPLES

Meal prepping doesn't need to be complicated. But the following guidelines can make it even easier.

START SIMPLY

An easy place to start is with readily available ingredients for simple recipes. To ease yourself in, focus on prepping a couple of meals a week at first, including a few staples and some basics like roasted chicken and vegetables, a hearty soup, or a breakfast casserole. As you get more comfortable with DASH and meal prep, you can expand the number of recipes you prep each week. In part 3, you'll find additional recipes that will inspire you to add even more variety to your preps.

USE INGREDIENTS WISELY

The beauty of meal prep is that you can use the same ingredients in different ways. When planning, consider not only your main ingredients but also what you use to flavor and add color to your meals. If you use onions and peppers in your morning frittata, plan to include them at lunch in a veggie wrap or in a soup. If you used orange juice for a marinade, consider adding oranges to your dinner salad. When choosing fresh herbs, remember that they can enhance flavor in almost any dish—sauces, marinades, salads, casseroles; don't ever let those herbs go to waste.

BE FLEXIBLE AND ADAPTABLE

As you start going through the different preps, you'll notice that we encourage variations, substitutions, and additions. We want you to feel comfortable substituting herbs in your seasonings, adding fruits or vegetables to your recipes, and even changing ingredients with some you might prefer or already have on hand. If your recipe calls for apples and you have pears that need to be used, feel free to swap them in. If you are making a stir-fry, preparing a casserole, roasting vegetables, or baking a frittata, leftover vegetables can always be added or substituted for additional flavor, color, and texture. When it comes to fruits and vegetables in DASH, more is better.

BE FOOD SAFETY SAVVY

Understanding the rules of food safety is essential when meal prepping. Although many leftovers may continue to *look* or smell okay, it is important to know how long you can safely store them. And even though most bacteria that make you ill will not grow in temperatures below 40°F, the bacteria that can cause food spoilage are still active at that temperature. Consider keeping your refrigerator between 35° to 38°F, an ideal temperature to allow an extra day or two of food storage. Freezing meals for later in the week is always a great option.

FOOD	REFRIGERATOR	FREEZER
COOKED POULTRY DISHES	3 to 4 days	4 to 6 months
COOKED FISH	3 to 4 days	4 to 6 months
COOKED MEAT DISHES	3 to 4 days	2 to 3 months
COOKED SALADS	3 to 5 days	Don't freeze
HARD-BOILED EGGS	1 week	Don't freeze
PREPARED EGG DISHES	3 to 4 days	2 to 3 months
SOUPS AND STEWS	3 to 4 days	2 to 3 months

Source: Food and Drug Administration Refrigerator & Freezer Storage Chart

CREATING YOUR DASH KITCHEN

Prepping your weekly meals involves some basic kitchen equipment, which you'll most likely already have on hand. The right tools make meal prepping an easier and more enjoyable process.

MUST-HAVES

Baking dishes: a plus if they have lids, since you can use them for cooking and storage

Blender: for smoothies, salad dressings, and soups

Colander: for draining pasta and washing fruits and vegetables

Cutting boards: at least two, one for meats and a separate one for vegetables

Fine-mesh sieve: especially good for draining fine grains, such as quinoa or rice

Food processor: to make blending sauces and ingredients effortless

Food thermometer: to ensure foods are cooked and reheated to safe temperatures

Knives: especially a chef's knife

Measuring cups and spoons: to make following recipes a snap

Muffin tin: for bite-size meals and snacks

Pasta pot: provides the depth you need to boil those noodles

Saucepans with lids: minimum of two different sizes

Sheet pan: also called a rimmed baking sheet; for easy sheet pan meals

Skillets: at least two—one large and one small or medium; ideally one should also be oven-safe

NICE-TO-HAVE

Air fryer: to transform some of your favorites into healthier-for-you options

Garlic press: an easier way to prep this magic ingredient

Immersion blender: makes it easy to blend soups right in the pot

Silicone baking mats: help keep your food from sticking, so no need for cooking spray

Spiralizer: for creative ways to use veggies

Zester/grater: for adding an extra layer of flavor

STORAGE ESSENTIALS

Once you are done prepping your meals, you'll need to store them properly. The last thing you want is to open Wednesday's lunch and find a soggy salad or a dry protein that's tough to eat. Here are the best storage practices that will ensure your meals maintain the highest quality possible.

GRAB-AND-GO CONTAINERS

Glass containers with airtight lids (single- and multi-compartment). These containers are simple and efficient. They are stackable, portable, and easy to take from the refrigerator to the freezer to the microwave to the dishwasher without a fuss. If you can find one with a reheating vent, that's a bonus. We strongly recommend having a variety of these handy containers. The single-compartment ones are great for salads, casseroles, and one-pot meals. They come in small (16-ounce), medium (24-ounce), and large (48-ounce) sizes. But when storing a meal with foods of different flavors and textures, having a multi-compartment container to separate them is ideal. They usually come in a 28-ounce size. The different-size compartments are also a great way to help you with portion control.

Mason jars (all sizes). These inexpensive containers are such a useful way to store your soups, salads, and sauces. They are glass and therefore microwave, dishwasher, and freezer friendly. Seek out BPA-free plastic lids to replace the included metal ones to keep these jars for long-term use.

Metal storage containers. These are great for foods or meals that do not require reheating, since they are not microwave-safe. Think salads, ready-to-eat snacks, and cold breakfast meals.

Mini condiment cups with lids. When packing your on-the-go meals, you often will find that textures create variety. To prevent your salad from deteriorating from the dressing or your granola turning to mush by the time you eat your parfait, you'll find these small cups to be just right for toppings, snacks, sauces, and more. These little plastic containers with snap-on lids come in a variety of sizes from 2 to 4 ounces. We find this type of storage to be more versatile than the dressing squeeze bottles.

Reusable silicone food bags. Make your fresh produce last longer with silicone food storage bags with airtight seals. These environment-friendly, waste-reducing bags can replace your sandwich- and half-gallon-size disposable bags. They come in a variety of colors and sizes, and many are even dishwasher-safe. (Yes, we know. We couldn't believe it either.)

Silicone collapsible food storage. These space-saving containers are not just stackable and easy to store but can also be used to reheat your food. The silicone material makes them BPA-free and microwave, refrigerator, and freezer friendly. (Many are even oven-safe.) When done, just place them in the dishwasher for easy cleanup.

REFRIGERATOR AND FREEZER BASICS

Be mindful of storage times. Cook poultry and fish within two days and red meats within three to five days of purchase. When storing raw meats in the refrigerator, keep them on the bottom shelf to prevent their liquids from contaminating fresh foods. If you're not going to cook them within those safe time spans, move poultry, fish, and meats to the freezer to extend their storage time. (See the storage chart on page 16.)

Don't delay refrigerator time. Once you have prepped your meals, it's essential to move your food to the refrigerator within two hours. You might consider placing bigger meals in shallow containers to let them cool a little faster.

Food storage labels. Although you think you'll remember when you prepared a meal and the last day it's safe to eat, you won't. Trust us when we say *label them*. There is no safer way to identify a meal's shelf life than by marking it with the date by which you should eat it, freeze it, or toss it.

THAWING AND REHEATING

You can thaw your frozen meals in one of three ways:

- In the refrigerator—the longest but safest route
- Under cold water—in a leakproof package to avoid water getting in the container
- In the microwave—place at 50 percent of defrost power to evenly defrost, then cook immediately

There are a few frozen meals that can be reheated without thawing—think casserole, soup, or stew. In these cases, use a saucepan, microwave, or even the oven. The reheating process is longer since you are starting from frozen, but it is completely appropriate from a food-safety perspective.

When reheating refrigerated meals, you can use the oven, microwave, or stovetop. Heat them until the internal temperature reaches 165°F. Always let the food rest for about five minutes before checking the temperature, since the temperature will rise several degrees in many foods from residual heat. For soups or warm sauces, ensure that you have brought them to a rolling boil. To maintain moisture and allow for even reheating, make sure your meals are covered, but only loosely, to allow for some venting.

ABOUT THE MEAL PREPS AND RECIPES

Our goal is to set you up for success and make sure you feel comfortable with meal prepping. That's why we're providing six weeks of progressive meal preps. Each meal prep provides meals for one person for five days. Why five days and not seven? Four to five days is how long most cooked foods last safely in the fridge. Many people use the other two days to prep meals for the following week, and/or enjoy a meal or two out. You'll notice that the weeks start simply, with just a couple of meals to prep, and then grow more complex later, adding recipes to include more variety. If you are ready for a bigger challenge, feel free to start your meal prepping a few weeks into the program, and save the simpler weeks for when you are tight on time.

Meal Prep 1: 1 breakfast, 2 lunches or dinners

Meal Prep 2: 1 breakfast, 2 lunches or dinners

Meal Prep 3: 1 breakfast, 3 lunches or dinners

Meal Prep 4: 1 breakfast, 3 lunches or dinners, 1 snack

Meal Prep 5: 1 breakfast, 3 lunches or dinners, 1 snack

Meal Prep 6: 2 breakfasts, 3 lunches or dinners, 1 snack

As you continue your DASH meal prep journey, you'll find an assortment of new recipes in part 3 that you can swap into your weekly rotation to add variety to your menu.

We've made sure that all the recipes included in this book are simple, with easy-to-find ingredients and step-by-step directions to help you prep meals like a pro. Every recipe also includes tips, variations, and substitution ideas that will allow you to make changes and keep your meals interesting week after week.

And, as registered dietitian nutritionists, we give you nutritional information at the end of each recipe. It includes the macro- and micronutrients you are looking for in DASH, such as protein, fiber, calcium, potassium, magnesium, and vitamin D. In addition, you'll find that the recipes have labels that will help you adapt your meals for certain allergies, sensitivities, or preferences—especially helpful when cooking for friends or family. Look for these labels:

- Dairy-Free

- Egg-Free

- Gluten-Free

- Nut-Free

- Vegetarian/Vegan

Quinoa and Avocado
Breakfast Bowls
Page 27

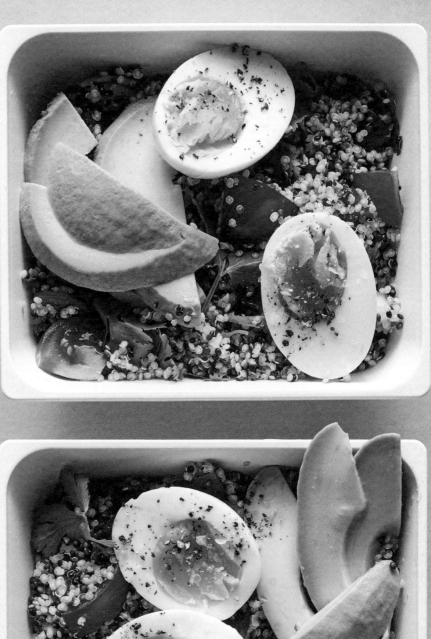
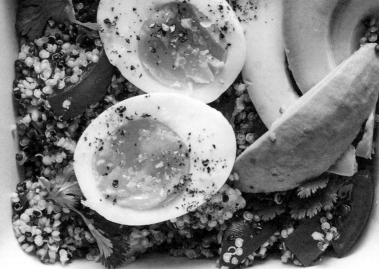

Crispy Fish Tacos with
Cilantro Slaw
Page 37

PART TWO

DASH MEAL PREPS

Many people are afraid that meal prepping means monotony, but we've put these preps together to showcase the incredible variety you can get with DASH. We'll share our secrets behind making our favorite foods efficiently—and a little more nutritiously. Remember, even though DASH was originally created for people with high blood pressure, it's a fantastic way for the whole family to eat. We'll bring the ideas. We hope *you'll* bring the willingness to embrace something new.

Meal Prep 1

Whether this is your first go at meal prep or you're a seasoned pro, we want you to succeed. Through this prep, we introduce you to the amazing flavor of herbs and spices you will continue to use while following DASH. This week, we give you a nontraditional breakfast recipe to start and energize your days. For your lunches and dinners, you'll find meals that are familiar and easy but with delicious flavors that make starting DASH a breeze.

RECIPE LIST

Quinoa and Avocado Breakfast Bowls

Sheet Pan Chicken and Roasted Vegetables

Barbecue Salmon and Crisp and Sweet Quinoa

SHOPPING LIST

Pantry items

- Black pepper
- Brown sugar
- Cayenne pepper
- Chili powder
- Cumin, ground
- Garlic powder
- Lemon juice
- Mustard powder
- Nonstick cooking spray
- Olive oil, extra-virgin
- Onion powder
- Paprika
- Quinoa (2 cups)

Produce

- Avocados (3)
- Bell peppers: red (1), yellow (1)
- Broccoli (1 small stalk)
- Chives, fresh (1 bunch)
- Cilantro, fresh (1 bunch)
- Cucumber (1 large)
- Dill (1 bunch)
- Garlic (1 clove)
- Green beans (12 ounces)
- Lemon (1)

- Lime (1)
- Mangos (2 large or 1 [15-ounce] can)
- Mushrooms (12 ounces, any kind)
- Onions, red (2 large)
- Parsley, fresh (2 bunches)
- Sweet potatoes (2 medium)
- Tomatoes (2 small)

Meat and seafood

- Chicken, boneless, skinless breasts (1 pound)
- Salmon, 5 (4-ounce) fillets

Dairy and eggs

- Eggs (5 large)
- Yogurt, Greek nonfat plain (6 ounces)

BE SURE YOU HAVE

- Condiment cups (5)
- Fine-mesh sieve
- Sheet pans (2)
- Storage containers (10 large)
- Storage containers (5 medium)

	BREAKFAST	LUNCH	DINNER
M	Quinoa and Avocado Breakfast Bowls	Sheet Pan Chicken and Roasted Vegetables	Barbecue Salmon and Crisp and Sweet Quinoa
T	Quinoa and Avocado Breakfast Bowls	Barbecue Salmon and Crisp and Sweet Quinoa	Sheet Pan Chicken and Roasted Vegetables
W	Quinoa and Avocado Breakfast Bowls	Sheet Pan Chicken and Roasted Vegetables	Barbecue Salmon and Crisp and Sweet Quinoa
TH	Quinoa and Avocado Breakfast Bowls	Barbecue Salmon and Crisp and Sweet Quinoa	Sheet Pan Chicken and Roasted Vegetables
F	Quinoa and Avocado Breakfast Bowls	Sheet Pan Chicken and Roasted Vegetables	Barbecue Salmon and Crisp and Sweet Quinoa

STEP-BY-STEP PREP:

1. Preheat the oven to 400°F.

2. Make the quinoa for the Quinoa and Avocado Breakfast Bowls (page 27) and the Crisp and Sweet Quinoa (page 107): Put 2 cups of quinoa (rinsed first if your brand has not been pre-rinsed) in a medium saucepan. Add 4 cups of water to the pan and bring to a boil. Cover, reduce the heat to a simmer, and cook for 15 to 20 minutes, or until all the water has absorbed and the grain is translucent and tender. Let sit for 5 minutes and fluff with a fork. Transfer the quinoa to a large bowl and set aside. Let cool for at least 5 minutes.

3. While the quinoa is cooking, put 5 eggs in a medium saucepan and add cold water to cover by 1 to 2 inches. (To make hard-boiled eggs easier to peel, purchase your eggs a week before cooking them. Two weeks is even better.)

4. Bring the water to a full rolling boil over high heat. Turn off the heat, but do not remove the saucepan from the hot burner. (If your stove has a burner that does not retain the heat, lower the temperature to low, simmer for a minute and then turn off the heat.) Cover and let sit for 10 to 12 minutes.

5. Run the eggs under cold water to quickly cool them (or put them in ice water). Peel and set aside.

6. While the quinoa and eggs are cooking and cooling, peel and prep all the vegetables, herbs, and fruit as directed in the individual recipes. Cut the chicken into bite-size cubes for the Sheet Pan Chicken and Roasted Vegetables (page 28). Make sure to use a separate cutting board for the raw chicken. Set all the ingredients aside.

7. Season and bake the chicken and vegetables, steps 2 to 7. Once the chicken and vegetables are done, remove from the oven and reduce the temperature to 350°F.

8. Season and bake the salmon (page 30), steps 2 and 3.

9. Assemble the breakfast bowls.

10. Assemble the Crisp and Sweet Quinoa.

11. Make the Greek Yogurt Dill Dressing (page 184).

QUINOA AND AVOCADO BREAKFAST BOWLS

Serves 5
Prep time: 10 minutes • **Cook time:** 25 minutes
DAIRY-FREE • GLUTEN-FREE • NUT-FREE • VEGETARIAN

Quinoa continues to reign as a superfood, a fitting description because it's jam-packed with nutritional benefits. It's an excellent source of fiber and provides plenty of the B vitamin folate, as well as iron and magnesium, minerals that can be difficult to find naturally in non-animal products. This ancient grain also ranks as one of the highest in protein, making it a top choice for those opting for a vegetarian or vegan lifestyle. The protein content of the quinoa and eggs, combined with the creaminess and fat in the avocado, will keep you satisfied until lunchtime. Pair with an orange or grapefruit for a nice twist on flavors and to add extra nutrition to your meal.

3¾ cups cooked quinoa

½ teaspoon onion powder

½ teaspoon freshly ground black pepper

½ teaspoon ground cumin

½ teaspoon garlic powder

1 tablespoon chopped fresh cilantro

2 small tomatoes, diced

½ large red onion, chopped

3 avocados, pitted, sliced, and coated with
   lemon juice

5 hard-boiled eggs, peeled and sliced

1. In a large bowl, season the cooked quinoa with the onion powder, pepper, cumin, and garlic powder. Add the cilantro, tomatoes, and onion. Mix well.
2. Divide the quinoa mix among 5 storage containers as a base for the breakfast bowl, then divide the avocados evenly into the bowls. Top each with a whole sliced egg.

- **Storage:** Seal airtight, and store in the refrigerator for up to 5 days. This dish may be served cold or warm. If warm is preferred, separate the egg and avocado from the quinoa mixture. Reheat the quinoa in the microwave for 1 minute. Then top with the egg and avocado.

- **Ingredient tip:** Frozen avocado cubes are readily available at your local grocer. Instead of adding fresh avocado from the start, add a few frozen pieces on top the night before, and they will have softened by breakfast time.

  Per Serving: Calories: 388; Total fat: 20g; Carbohydrates: 40g; Fiber: 10g; Protein: 15g; Calcium: 72mg; Vitamin D: 41 IU; Potassium: 812mg; Magnesium: 124mg; Sodium: 90mg

SHEET PAN CHICKEN AND ROASTED VEGETABLES

Serves 5
Prep time: 15 minutes • **Cook time:** 30 minutes
DAIRY-FREE • EGG-FREE • GLUTEN-FREE • NUT-FREE

One-pan meals are a favorite because of their convenience and simplicity. What we love about this recipe is that you can add additional vegetables to the mix. Try this with cauliflower, eggplant, or zucchini. The more color and variety, the better it is for you.

Nonstick cooking spray

1 teaspoon garlic powder

1 teaspoon freshly ground black pepper

1 teaspoon ground cumin

1 teaspoon paprika

2 medium sweet potatoes, cubed

3 tablespoons extra-virgin olive oil, divided

1 pound boneless, skinless chicken breasts, cut into small pieces

1 small broccoli stalk, cut into florets (about 2 cups)

1 red bell pepper, cut into 1-inch pieces

1 yellow bell pepper, cut into 1-inch pieces

1½ cups sliced mushrooms

1½ cups green beans, cut into 1-inch pieces

½ large red onion, cut into 1-inch chunks

Juice of 1 lemon

2 tablespoons chopped fresh parsley

1. Preheat the oven to 400°F. Line 2 sheet pans with aluminum foil and coat with nonstick cooking spray.
2. In a small bowl, combine the garlic powder, black pepper, cumin, and paprika.
3. In a large bowl, toss the sweet potatoes with 1 tablespoon of oil. Season with 1 teaspoon of the mixed spices. Toss until well coated.
4. Spread the sweet potatoes in a single layer on a sheet pan and roast for 10 minutes. The sweet potatoes should still be too firm to eat. Keep the oven on and set the pan aside.
5. In the same large bowl, toss together the chicken, broccoli, red bell pepper, yellow bell pepper, mushrooms, green beans, onion, the remaining 2 tablespoons of oil, the lemon juice, and the remaining spice mixture. Toss until everything is well coated.
6. Divide the sweet potatoes, chicken, and vegetables between the sheet pans, distributing everything evenly in a single layer.

7. Bake for 15 to 20 minutes, or until the vegetables are tender and the chicken is cooked through with no pink in the center.
8. Sprinkle everything with the parsley, then divide the contents of the sheet pans evenly into 5 storage containers.

- **Storage:** Seal airtight, and store in the refrigerator for up to 5 days. To heat, vent the lid slightly, and reheat in the microwave for 2 minutes.

  Per Serving: Calories: 305; Total fat: 17g; Carbohydrates: 22g; Fiber: 4.5g; Protein: 22g; Calcium: 63mg; Vitamin D: 4 IU; Potassium: 726mg; Magnesium: 58mg; Sodium: 85mg

BARBECUE SALMON AND CRISP AND SWEET QUINOA

Serves 5

Prep time: 15 minutes • **Cook time:** 20 minutes

EGG-FREE • GLUTEN-FREE • NUT-FREE

Salmon is extremely rich in omega-3 fatty acids, which is beneficial to heart health when consumed at least twice a week. To add a twist to this fish, we seasoned it with a dry barbecue rub. Don't be surprised if even non-fish lovers find it delicious. We've paired the salmon with quinoa salad dressed with a Greek Yogurt Dill Dressing (page 184) to give it a little extra zing.

Nonstick cooking spray

¼ cup packed brown sugar

2 teaspoons garlic powder

2 teaspoons onion powder

1 teaspoon mustard powder

½ teaspoon chili powder (optional)

1 teaspoon paprika

1 teaspoon freshly ground black pepper

¼ teaspoon cayenne pepper

5 (4-ounce) salmon fillets, skinless

Crisp and Sweet Quinoa (page 107)

Greek Yogurt Dill Dressing (page 184) or
    1 cup store-bought

1. Preheat the oven to 350°F. Coat a sheet pan with cooking spray.
2. In a small bowl, combine the brown sugar, garlic powder, onion powder, mustard powder, chili powder (if using), paprika, black pepper, and cayenne pepper. Season the salmon fillets with this rub.
3. Place the salmon on the prepared sheet pan and bake for 12 to 15 minutes, or until the salmon is cooked through.
4. Place a salmon fillet and 1¼ cups of the quinoa into each of 5 storage containers. Divide the dressing among 5 condiment cups.

- **Storage:** Seal airtight, and refrigerate for up to 5 days. Salmon may be eaten cold or hot. To reheat, heat the salmon fillet for 90 seconds in the microwave. Quinoa salad should be served cold and drizzled with dressing.

- **Substitution tip:** You can use 1 tablespoon of Dijon mustard or yellow mustard instead of the mustard powder.

- **Cooking tip:** Avoid overcooking the salmon. To check for doneness, gently pull at the top of the fillet with a fork. If it pulls apart in moist flakes, it's done.

Per Serving: Calories: 477; Total fat: 17g; Carbohydrates: 48g; Fiber: 5g; Protein: 36g; Calcium: 120mg; Vitamin D: 282 IU; Potassium: 1,190mg; Magnesium: 133mg; Sodium: 83mg

Meal Prep 2

This week, we emphasize flexibility and variety. Many of the recipes that follow focus on cooking from scratch. Why? You control the amount of salt, sugar, and fats in your food. It also allows you to select the right portion size for each meal. Fresh ingredients mean a little more work, but we promise that the taste and nutrition are worth the extra time. You'll also make a granola that stores easily for up to a month. And we'll go heavy on nutrient-rich and satisfying fruits, vegetables, and whole grains to make your DASH plate.

RECIPE LIST

Cinnamon-Berry Greek Yogurt Parfaits with Super-Simple Granola

Crispy Fish Tacos with Cilantro Slaw

Skirt Steak Six-Layer Salad

SHOPPING LIST

Pantry items

- Almonds, slivered (¾ cup)
- Black pepper
- Bread crumbs (½ cup)
- Cinnamon, ground
- Flour, whole wheat (¼ cup)
- Honey
- Lemon pepper

- Nonstick cooking spray
- Oats, rolled (2 cups)
- Olive oil, extra-virgin
- Salt
- Vanilla extract
- Vinegar, apple cider
- Walnuts, chopped (½ cup)

Produce

- Apple, green (1)
- Blueberries (1 pint)
- Cabbage (1 small head)
- Chives (1 bunch)
- Cilantro (1 bunch)

- Corn (2 ears)
- Cucumbers (2 medium)
- Dill (1 bunch)
- Garlic (3 cloves)
- Jalapeño pepper (1)

- Lettuce, romaine (1 head)
- Limes (3)
- Onions, red (2 medium)
- Parsley (1 bunch)

Meat and seafood

- Cod fillets (1 pound)
- Skirt steak (1 pound)

Dairy and eggs

- Egg (1 large)
- Milk, 1% (1 ounce)

Other

- Tortillas, corn (10)

- Raspberries (1 pint)
- Strawberries (1 pint)
- Tomatoes, grape (1 pint)

- Queso fresco (5 ounces)
- Yogurt, Greek nonfat plain (6 cups)

BE SURE YOU HAVE

- Divided storage containers (5 large)
- Oven-safe skillet (1)
- Resealable bag (1)

- Sheet pans (2)
- Storage containers (5 large)
- Storage containers (5 medium)

	BREAKFAST	LUNCH	DINNER
M	Cinnamon-Berry Greek Yogurt Parfaits with Super-Simple Granola	Crispy Fish Tacos with Cilantro Slaw	Skirt Steak Six-Layer Salad
T	Cinnamon-Berry Greek Yogurt Parfaits with Super-Simple Granola	Skirt Steak Six-Layer Salad	Crispy Fish Tacos with Cilantro Slaw
W	Cinnamon-Berry Greek Yogurt Parfaits with Super-Simple Granola	Crispy Fish Tacos with Cilantro Slaw	Skirt Steak Six-Layer Salad
TH	Cinnamon-Berry Greek Yogurt Parfaits with Super-Simple Granola	Skirt Steak Six-Layer Salad	Crispy Fish Tacos with Cilantro Slaw
F	Cinnamon-Berry Greek Yogurt Parfaits with Super-Simple Granola	Crispy Fish Tacos with Cilantro Slaw	Skirt Steak Six-Layer Salad

STEP-BY-STEP PREP:

1. Finely chop the fresh herbs for the Crispy Fish Tacos with Cilantro Slaw (page 37) and Skirt Steak Six-Layer Salad (page 39).

2. Marinate the skirt steak, step 1 of the skirt steak recipe.

3. If making the Super-Simple Granola (page 91), preheat the oven to 350°F.

4. Assemble and bake the granola, steps 2 and 3.

5. Flavor the yogurt for the Cinnamon-Berry Greek Yogurt Parfaits with Super-Simple Granola (page 36), step 1.

6. If not making homemade granola, position racks in the upper and lower thirds of the oven and preheat the oven to 450°F. Preheat the skillet for the skirt steak on the upper rack.

7. Bake the fish, steps 1 to 3 of the fish taco recipe.

8. Take out the fish. Carefully remove the preheated skillet and cook the skirt steak, step 4 of the skirt steak recipe.

9. Meanwhile, chop the vegetables for the five-layer salad.

10. Make the Greek Yogurt Dill Dressing (page 184).

11. Make the cilantro slaw for the tacos. Assemble the tacos.

12. Assemble the skirt steak salads.

13. Assemble the yogurt and granola parfaits.

CINNAMON-BERRY GREEK YOGURT PARFAITS WITH SUPER-SIMPLE GRANOLA

Serves 5
Prep time: 10 minutes • **Cook time:** 25 minutes (if making granola)
EGG-FREE • VEGETARIAN • GLUTEN-FREE OPTION (SEE TIP)

Start your morning with a *dash* of natural sweetness and protein. Greek yogurt is a DASH superstar. Depending on the brand, it can offer up to 17 grams of high-quality protein per serving. It also has other essential nutrients—including calcium, phosphorus, riboflavin, vitamin B_{12}, and pantothenic acid—to help build and maintain your body, as well as zinc, to ensure your immune system is working properly. When buying yogurt, check the label for "live and active cultures," which means the yogurt contains good bacteria that benefit your digestive system.

---

5 cups nonfat plain Greek yogurt

1 tablespoon ground cinnamon

10 tablespoons Super-Simple Granola (page 91) or store-bought

2½ cups fresh berries (any kind), sliced if large

1. In a medium bowl, stir together the Greek yogurt and cinnamon.
2. Evenly divide the yogurt among 5 storage containers. Distribute 2 tablespoons of granola and ½ cup of fresh berries to each container.

- **Storage:** Keep the storage containers in the refrigerator for up to 5 days.

- **Variations:** Feel free to swap in or add pecans, cashews, or pistachios to the granola, and consider changing the fresh fruit for a more seasonal blend: citrus in the winter or peaches in the summer.

- **Gluten-free option:** To make this gluten-free, purchase certified gluten-free oats.

Per Serving: Calories: 265; Total fat: 7g; Carbohydrates: 26g; Fiber: 6g; Protein: 27g; Calcium: 313mg; Vitamin D: 0 IU; Potassium: 499mg; Magnesium: 58mg; Sodium: 113mg

CRISPY FISH TACOS WITH CILANTRO SLAW

Serves 5
Prep time: 20 minutes • **Cook time:** 15 minutes
NUT-FREE OPTION (SEE TIP)

We've taken a better-for-you approach with this dish by baking instead of frying the fish and adding plenty of vegetables (but without sacrificing taste). Combining the protein with a whole-grain tortilla and a crunchy slaw helps you get more DASH foods on your plate.

FOR THE FISH

Nonstick cooking spray

¼ cup whole wheat flour

1 large egg, beaten

2 tablespoons 1% milk

½ cup dried unseasoned bread crumbs

¼ cup slivered almonds

¼ teaspoon lemon pepper

1 teaspoon chopped fresh parsley

1 pound fresh or (thawed) frozen skinless cod, divided into 5 (about 3-ounce) fillets

1 tablespoon extra-virgin olive oil

FOR THE CILANTRO SLAW

5 cups chopped cabbage

1 medium red onion, diced

1 medium green apple, julienned

1 jalapeño pepper, diced

¼ cup chopped fresh cilantro

¼ cup extra-virgin olive oil

Juice of 2 small limes

¼ teaspoon salt

FOR THE TACOS

10 corn tortillas

5 ounces queso fresco

Continued ❯

TO MAKE THE FISH

1. Preheat the oven to 450°F. Coat a sheet pan with cooking spray or line with a silicone baking mat.
2. Line up 3 shallow bowls or dishes. Put the flour in the first bowl. In the second, whisk together the egg and milk. In the third, combine the bread crumbs, almonds, lemon pepper, and parsley. Coat each cod fillet first in the flour, then the egg wash, and then the bread crumb mixture. Place on the prepared sheet pan and drizzle with the oil.
3. Bake the cod for about 15 minutes, or until crisp and just cooked through.

TO MAKE THE CILANTRO SLAW

4. In a large bowl, combine the cabbage, onion, apple, jalapeño pepper, and cilantro. Toss to mix.
5. In a small bowl, whisk together the oil, lime juice, and salt. Add to the slaw and mix.

TO MAKE THE TACOS

6. Slice the cod fillets.
7. In 5 divided storage containers, place the sliced fillets on 2 tortillas in one partition, and the cilantro slaw in the other. Add ½ ounce of crumbled queso fresco to each taco.

- **Storage:** Seal airtight, and store the containers in the refrigerator for up to 5 days. Reheat the fish for 1 to 2 minutes in the microwave. Place on top of the tortillas, and add the slaw.

- **Cooking tip:** For fresh herbs like cilantro and parsley, grab the stem and hold your knife at an angle while chopping; this gets the leaves off while leaving the stem behind.

- **Nut-free option:** Leave the almonds out of the coating.

Per Serving: Calories: 479; Total fat: 26g; Carbohydrates: 37g; Fiber: 6g; Protein: 27g; Calcium: 255mg; Vitamin D: 66 IU; Potassium: 503mg; Magnesium: 70mg; Sodium: 450mg

SKIRT STEAK SIX-LAYER SALAD

Serves 5
Prep time: 20 minutes, plus 30 minutes to marinate • **Cook time:** 15 minutes
EGG-FREE • GLUTEN-FREE • NUT-FREE

The flavor secret of this recipe is a robust marinade and a little bit of time. To cut down on prep time, place the steak in the refrigerator the night before to marinate. If you don't have time, however, don't worry. Even 30 minutes can add fantastic flavor.

FOR THE STEAK

1 pound skirt steak

¼ cup extra-virgin olive oil

2 tablespoons chopped fresh parsley

Juice of 1 lime

2 garlic cloves, minced

1 teaspoon freshly ground black pepper

Nonstick cooking spray

FOR THE SALAD

10 tablespoons Greek Yogurt Dill Dressing
   (page 184) or store-bought

1 head romaine lettuce, chopped

1 cup grape tomatoes, halved

2 medium cucumbers, diced

1 medium red onion, diced

1 cup fresh corn kernels

TO MAKE THE STEAK

1. In a large resealable bag, combine the skirt steak, oil, parsley, lime juice, garlic, and pepper. Marinate for 30 minutes or up to 24 hours.
2. Preheat the oven to 450°F.
3. Place a large oven-safe sauté pan or skillet in the oven and preheat for 30 minutes.
4. Remove the pan from the oven and coat lightly with nonstick cooking spray. Place the skirt steak in the pan and return it to the oven for 6 to 9 minutes, depending on how rare you would like the meat. Flip and return for 3 to 4½ minutes. Let rest for 5 minutes before slicing across the grain of the meat. For a medium-rare steak, the internal temperature should reach 135°F.

Continued ❯

SKIRT STEAK SIX-LAYER SALAD   *Continued*

5. Evenly divide the dressing on the bottom of 5 storage containers.

6. Layer the steak first, then the lettuce, tomatoes, cucumbers, onion, and corn.

- **Storage:** Seal airtight, and store the containers in the refrigerator for up to 5 days.

- **Substitution tip:** The Simple Green Salad (page 118) is another great base option for the steak. Add Lemon Vinaigrette (page 183) for some extra tang.

  Per Serving: Calories: 293; Total fat: 15g; Carbohydrates: 17g; Fiber: 4.5g; Protein: 26g; Calcium: 92mg; Vitamin D: 3 IU; Potassium: 785mg; Magnesium: 60mg; Sodium: 67mg

Meal Prep 3

By now, your meal prep confidence should be growing, and along with it, the number of recipes you'll use; it increases to four this week. For this prep, we want you to become comfortable using canned and frozen ingredients when needed. Many canned beans, sauces, and vegetables are available in no-salt-added or low-sodium varieties. Frozen vegetables are picked at their peak and flash frozen to maintain nutritional benefits without added preservatives. Learning when and how to substitute these in a recipe will help you improvise when you are running low on an ingredient or unable to find it at the market.

RECIPE LIST

Veggie Frittata

Vegetable Wraps with Minestrone Soup

Rosemary and Lemon Pepper Pork with Spinach-Citrus Salad

Sweet Glazed Chicken, Rosemary Potatoes, and Green Beans

SHOPPING LIST

Canned and bottled items

- Kidney beans, no-salt-added
  (1 [8-ounce] can)
- Navy beans, no-salt-added
  (1 [8-ounce] can)
- Tomatoes, diced, no-salt-added
  (1 [8-ounce] can)
- Tomato sauce, no-salt-added
  (1 [5-ounce] can)

Pantry items

- Black pepper
- Chicken stock, unsalted (2½ cups)
- Cumin, ground
- Dried basil
- Dried oregano leaves
- Dried parsley
- Dried rosemary
- Garlic powder
- Honey
- Macaroni, whole wheat elbow (⅔ cup)
- Mustard, Dijon
- Olive oil, extra-virgin

- Onion powder
- Paprika
- Salt
- Sugar, brown (3 tablespoons)
- Sunflower seeds, unsalted, roasted (9 tablespoons)
- Vinegar, apple cider

Produce

- Baby spinach (8½ cups)
- Bell peppers: green (1 small), red (1 medium)
- Carrots (2 large)
- Celery (2 stalks)
- Cilantro (1 bunch)
- Garlic (8 cloves)
- Green beans (¾ pound)
- Lemons (3)
- Mushrooms, any kind (6 ounces)
- Onions: red (2 medium), yellow (1 medium)
- Oranges (4 medium)
- Parsley (1 bunch)
- Potatoes, red (1¼ pounds, small)
- Tomato (1 large)

Meat

- Chicken, 3 (3-ounce) boneless, skinless breasts
- Pork, 4 (4-ounce) boneless center-cut chops

Dairy and eggs

- Cheddar cheese, shredded, reduced-fat (½ cup)
- Cottage cheese, low-fat (4 ounces)
- Eggs (7 large)

Other

- Tortillas or wraps, whole wheat, 10-inch (3)

BE SURE YOU HAVE

- Divided storage containers (8)
- Fine-mesh sieve
- Grater
- Oven-safe skillet (1)
- Resealable bags (3)
- Sheet pan (1)
- Storage containers (7 large, divided)
- Storage containers (8 medium)
- Thermometer
- Toothpicks
- Zester

	BREAKFAST	LUNCH	DINNER
M	Veggie Frittata	Vegetable Wraps with Minestrone Soup	Rosemary and Lemon Pepper Pork with Spinach-Citrus Salad
T	Veggie Frittata	Rosemary and Lemon Pepper Pork with Spinach-Citrus Salad	Sweet Glazed Chicken, Rosemary Potatoes, and Green Beans
W	Veggie Frittata	Sweet Glazed Chicken, Rosemary Potatoes, and Green Beans	Vegetable Wraps with Minestrone Soup
TH	Veggie Frittata	Rosemary and Lemon Pepper Pork with Spinach-Citrus Salad	Sweet Glazed Chicken, Rosemary Potatoes, and Green Beans
F	Veggie Frittata	Vegetable Wraps with Minestrone Soup	Rosemary and Lemon Pepper Pork with Spinach-Citrus Salad

STEP-BY-STEP PREP:

1. Preheat the oven to 425°F.

2. Prepare, bake, and store the Veggie Frittata (page 44), steps 2 to 5.

3. Change the oven setting to broil (with the rack about 4 inches from the top).

4. Meanwhile, make and assemble the vegetable wraps (page 49), steps 1 to 4.

5. Make the dressing and salad and broil the pork for the Rosemary and Lemon Pepper Pork with Spinach-Citrus Salad (page 45), steps 1 to 7.

6. When done, change the oven setting to bake at 400°F.

7. Cook the chicken, roast the potatoes, and cook the greens beans for Sweet Glazed Chicken, Rosemary Potatoes, and Green Beans (page 47), steps 1 to 9.

8. Make the minestrone soup (page 50), steps 5 to 8.

VEGGIE FRITTATA

Serves 5
Prep time: 10 minutes • **Cook time:** 15 minutes
GLUTEN-FREE • NUT-FREE • VEGETARIAN

Eating vegetables at breakfast is not intuitive. With this delicious frittata recipe, you will be surprised at how easy it is to get a full serving of veggies in your first meal of the day. This also makes for an excellent crowd-pleaser and a great weekend brunch option.

7 large eggs
2 garlic cloves, minced
¼ teaspoon onion powder
1 teaspoon dried oregano
1 teaspoon dried rosemary
½ teaspoon freshly ground black pepper

1 large tomato, chopped
1 small green bell pepper, chopped
½ medium red onion, chopped
½ cup shredded reduced-fat Cheddar
    cheese, divided
1½ teaspoons extra-virgin olive oil

1. Preheat the oven to 425°F.
2. In a large bowl, whisk together the eggs, garlic, onion powder, oregano, rosemary, and black pepper. Add the tomato, bell pepper, onion, and ¼ cup of Cheddar cheese. Whisk to combine.
3. Coat an oven-safe medium skillet with the oil. Pour in the mixture and sprinkle with the remaining ¼ cup of cheese.
4. Bake for about 15 minutes, or until the eggs are fully cooked.
5. Slice into 5 wedges and place in storage containers or reusable bags.

- **Storage:** Seal airtight, and refrigerate the containers or bags for up to 5 days. To reheat, microwave on high for 45 seconds.

- **Ingredient tip:** To make this a complete DASH meal, serve with fruit and Greek yogurt.

  Per Serving: Calories: 162; Total fat: 10g; Carbohydrates: 5g; Fiber: 1g; Protein: 13g; Calcium: 159mg; Vitamin D: 59 IU; Potassium: 249mg; Magnesium: 21mg; Sodium: 185mg

ROSEMARY AND LEMON PEPPER PORK WITH SPINACH-CITRUS SALAD

Serves 4

Prep time: 25 minutes • **Cook time:** 10 minutes

DAIRY-FREE • EGG-FREE • GLUTEN-FREE • NUT-FREE

Center-cut chops are a lean and delicious way to incorporate flavorful pork into your diet. They provide an excellent source of protein to keep you satisfied, as well as potassium, which keeps them DASH friendly. The combination of citrus and rosemary gives this dish a flavorful pop.

FOR THE SALAD

Juice of ½ orange

1½ tablespoons apple cider vinegar

2 tablespoons extra-virgin olive oil

2 teaspoons Dijon mustard

2 teaspoons honey

¼ teaspoon freshly ground black pepper

2 teaspoons chopped fresh cilantro

6 cups baby spinach

1 small onion, thinly sliced

1½ oranges, peeled and sliced or separated into sections

¼ cup unsalted roasted sunflower seeds

FOR THE PORK

2 garlic cloves, minced

Zest of 2 lemons

Juice of 1 lemon

1 teaspoon dried rosemary

4 (4-ounce) boneless center-cut pork chops

1 teaspoon freshly ground black pepper

½ teaspoon salt

TO MAKE THE SALAD

1. In a small bowl, mix together the orange juice, vinegar, oil, mustard, honey, pepper, and cilantro. Set aside.
2. In a large bowl, toss together the spinach, onion, oranges, and sunflower seeds. Set aside.

Continued ❯

TO MAKE THE PORK

3. Position a rack 4 inches from the heating element and preheat the broiler.
4. In a small bowl, mash the garlic with the back of a spoon to make a paste. Add the lemon zest, lemon juice, and rosemary and stir.
5. Rub the pork chops on both sides with the paste. Sprinkle with the pepper and salt.
6. Place the pork chops on a broiler pan and broil for 3 to 5 minutes on each side until barely pink in the center. The center of the chop should read 145°F.
7. Divide the pork and salad into separate storage containers. Store the dressing in condiment cups.

- **Storage:** Seal airtight, and refrigerate for up to 5 days. Reheat the pork by venting the lid and microwaving for 90 seconds. Add the dressing to the salad just before serving.

- **Substitution tip:** You can use a 10-ounce can of mandarin oranges (drained) and 1½ ounces of orange juice if fresh oranges are not available.

- **Cooking tip:** This recipe also works great on a grill; use medium-high heat and grill the pork for 3 to 5 minutes per side.

  Per Serving: Calories: 334; Total fat: 18g; Carbohydrates: 18g; Fiber: 4.5g; Protein: 26g; Calcium: 147mg; Vitamin D: 0 IU; Potassium: 529mg; Magnesium: 91mg; Sodium: 464mg

SWEET GLAZED CHICKEN, ROSEMARY POTATOES, AND GREEN BEANS

Serves 3
Prep time: 10 minutes • **Cook time:** 25 minutes
DAIRY-FREE • EGG-FREE • GLUTEN-FREE • NUT-FREE

This recipe is a favorite of Maria-Paula's family. There's no fuss at dinnertime when preparing this easy and balanced meal. What she loves most is that it easily doubles for those nights when unexpected guests arrive, but also freezes well if too much is left. Best of all, it all stores together and can be reheated at the same time.

FOR THE CHICKEN

3 tablespoons brown sugar

½ teaspoon freshly ground black pepper

¼ teaspoon ground cumin

¼ teaspoon paprika

½ teaspoon garlic powder

3 (4-ounce) thin-sliced chicken breast cutlets

1 tablespoon extra-virgin olive oil

FOR THE POTATOES AND BEANS

1½ pounds small red potatoes, quartered

3 tablespoons extra-virgin olive oil, divided

¾ teaspoon freshly ground black pepper, divided

2 garlic cloves, minced

1 tablespoon dried rosemary

1½ cups water

12 ounces green beans, trimmed

Juice of 1 lemon

1½ tablespoons unsalted roasted sunflower seeds

TO MAKE THE CHICKEN

1. In a small bowl, stir together the brown sugar, pepper, cumin, paprika, and garlic powder.
2. Coat both sides of each chicken breast with this mixture.
3. In a large skillet, heat the oil over medium heat. Make sure the bottom of the skillet is coated. Add the chicken and cook for about 5 minutes on each side, or until it is no longer pink on the inside and the glaze is deep brown.

Continued ❯

TO MAKE THE POTATOES AND BEANS

4. Preheat the oven to 400°F.

5. In a large bowl, toss the potatoes with 2 tablespoons of oil, ½ teaspoon of pepper, the garlic, and rosemary.

6. Spread the potatoes in a single layer on a sheet pan.

7. Bake for 10 to 15 minutes, flip them, and bake for an additional 10 minutes if you want them a little browner and crispier.

8. Meanwhile, in a medium saucepan, bring the water to a boil. Add the green beans, cover, and cook for 4 to 5 minutes, or until tender.

9. Drain the beans and transfer to a large bowl with room to toss with seasonings. Add the lemon juice and the remaining 1 tablespoon of oil and ¼ teaspoon of pepper.

10. In 3 storage containers, preferably with partitions, place a chicken cutlet in each, then divide the potatoes and green beans evenly among the containers. Sprinkle ½ tablespoon of sunflower seeds on top of each serving of green beans.

- **Storage:** Seal airtight, and store in the refrigerator for up to 5 days or in the freezer for 2 to 3 months. To reheat, vent the lid slightly, and microwave for 2 minutes. To reheat from frozen, vent the container, and reheat in the microwave for 3 minutes.

- **Substitution tip:** Frozen green beans can be used in place of fresh. Cook them according to the package directions, and season as the recipe directs.

Per Serving: Calories: 546; Total fat: 23g; Carbohydrates: 57g; Fiber: 8.5g; Protein: 31g; Calcium: 113mg; Vitamin D: 3 IU; Potassium: 1,557mg; Magnesium: 107mg; Sodium: 107mg

VEGETABLE WRAPS WITH MINESTRONE SOUP

Serves 3
Prep time: 25 minutes • **Cook time:** 20 minutes
EGG-FREE • NUT-FREE • VEGETARIAN

This meal combines both cool and hot temperatures and a mix of light and hearty ingredients. Though simple, this wrap and soup combo will leave you feeling satisfied for hours. It may look like a lot of ingredients, but we promise it is simple. Plus, the variety of vegetables, whole grains, and beans are powerful sources of fiber to help you meet your daily nutritional needs.

FOR THE WRAPS

½ cup low-fat cottage cheese

Zest of 1 lemon

¼ teaspoon freshly ground black pepper

2 teaspoons dried oregano

3 (10-inch) whole wheat tortillas or wraps

1 cup spinach leaves

1 large carrot, shredded

½ red bell pepper, thinly sliced

½ medium red onion, thinly sliced

6 ounces mushrooms, thinly sliced

3 tablespoons unsalted roasted
   sunflower seeds

FOR THE SOUP

1½ tablespoons extra-virgin olive oil

1 large carrot, diced

½ medium red onion, chopped

2 celery stalks, chopped

2 garlic cloves, minced

2½ cups unsalted chicken stock, divided

1 (5-ounce) can no-salt-added tomato sauce

1 (8-ounce) can no-salt-added navy beans,
   drained and rinsed

1 (8-ounce) can no-salt-added kidney beans,
   drained and rinsed

1 (8-ounce) can no-salt-added diced tomatoes

1½ cups chopped spinach

2 teaspoons dried basil

2 teaspoons dried parsley

1 teaspoon dried oregano

1 teaspoon onion powder

1 teaspoon freshly ground black pepper

⅔ cup elbow macaroni

TO MAKE THE WRAPS

1. In a medium bowl, combine the cottage cheese, lemon zest, black pepper, and oregano.
2. Spread the mixture onto the tortillas, leaving a 1-inch border around the edges.

Continued ❯

3. Layer the spinach leaves on top of the dressing. Add the carrot, bell pepper, onion, and mushrooms to the centers of the tortillas. Sprinkle with the sunflower seeds.
4. Fold up the bottoms, then fold in the sides and roll like a burrito without letting the contents spill out. You may use a toothpick to secure. If desired, cut in half.

TO MAKE THE SOUP

5. In a medium saucepan, heat the oil over medium heat. Add the carrot, onion, and celery and cook for 3 minutes. Add the garlic and sauté for another minute.
6. Pour in 1 cup of chicken stock, the tomato sauce, navy beans, and kidney beans. Mix well. Add the diced tomatoes, spinach, basil, parsley, oregano, onion powder, and pepper. Bring to a boil over high heat, then reduce the heat to a simmer, cover, and cook for 15 minutes. Remove from the heat.
7. In a small saucepan, bring the remaining 1½ cups of chicken stock to a boil and add the macaroni. Cook uncovered for 6 to 8 minutes, or until the macaroni is tender. Drain and set aside to cool for 5 minutes.
8. Add the cooked macaroni to the soup and combine.
9. Store the wraps and soup separately.

- **Storage:** Seal airtight, and store in the refrigerator for up to 5 days. The soup can be frozen for up to 1 month. Wraps can be served cold. To reheat the soup, vent the lid, and microwave for 2 minutes.

- **Ingredient tip:** An easy way to use extra tortillas from the package is to make some chips. Simply cut them into 4 wedges, and bake at 350°F for 5 to 8 minutes. Make more of the cottage cheese mixture you made for the wraps, and spread some on the chips.

  Per Serving: Calories: 549; Total fat: 15g; Carbohydrates: 84g; Fiber: 30g; Protein: 36g; Calcium: 351mg; Vitamin D: 2 IU; Potassium: 1,500mg; Magnesium: 119mg; Sodium: 770mg

Meal Prep 4

By now, you're on your way to becoming a meal prep master. This week gets a little more intense with five meals to prep. We'll give DASH makeovers to some of your favorite foods and offer some budget-saving tips. We take a traditional Waldorf salad and add a bit of protein with a flavorful cheese and seasoned chicken. We make over ordinary spaghetti and meatballs with a kid-friendly turkey option, homemade sauce, and whole wheat pasta—an easy way to get more potassium and magnesium, which help lower blood pressure and repair and restore muscles. It also includes vitamin C to boost immunity.

RECIPE LIST

Baked Egg, Spinach, and Tomato Cups

Waldorf Salad with Perfectly Poached Chicken

Basil and Pine Nut–Topped Sole with Apple Caprese Salad

Turkey Meatballs with Whole Wheat Penne in Simple Tomato Sauce

Fruit and Nut Trail Mix

SHOPPING LIST

Pantry items

- Almonds, unsalted (¼ cup)
- Bay leaf
- Black pepper
- Bread crumbs (½ cup)
- Chicken stock, unsalted (6 cups)
- Dark chocolate chips (¼ cup)
- Dried apricot (¼ cup)
- Dried cranberries (¼ cup)
- Herbes de Provence
- Honey

- Maple syrup
- Nonstick cooking spray
- Olive oil, extra-virgin
- Pasta, penne, whole wheat (8 ounces)
- Pine nuts (3 tablespoons)
- Red pepper flakes
- Salt
- Vinegar, balsamic
- Walnuts, chopped (½ cup)

Produce

- Apples, Gala (4 medium)
- Basil (1 bunch)
- Celery (4 stalks)
- Chives (1 bunch)
- Garlic (6 cloves)
- Grapes, seedless (1 cup)
- Lemon (1)
- Parsley (1 bunch)
- Spinach (6½ cups)
- Tomatoes (3 medium)
- Tomatoes, grape (2 pints)

Meat and seafood

- Chicken, 2 (8-ounce) boneless, skinless breasts
- Sole, 3 (4-ounce) fillets
- Turkey, ground (1 pound)

Dairy and eggs

- Cheddar cheese, shredded, reduced-fat (2½ ounces)
- Eggs (11 large)
- Feta cheese (2 tablespoons)
- Milk, 1% (¼ cup)
- Mozzarella cheese (3 ounces)
- Parmesan cheese, grated (½ cup)
- Yogurt, Greek nonfat plain (½ cup)

BE SURE YOU HAVE

- Condiment cups (8)
- Muffin tin (1)
- Paper liners or silicone muffin liners (optional)
- Sheet pan (1)
- Silicone baking mat (optional)
- Storage containers (8 large)
- Storage containers (13 medium)
- Storage containers (5 small)
- Thermometer

	BREAKFAST	LUNCH	DINNER	SNACK
M	Baked Egg, Spinach, and Tomato Cups	Turkey Meatballs with Whole Wheat Penne in Simple Tomato Sauce	Waldorf Salad with Perfectly Poached Chicken	Fruit and Nut Trail Mix
T	Baked Egg, Spinach, and Tomato Cups	Basil and Pine Nut–Topped Sole with Apple Caprese Salad	Turkey Meatballs with Whole Wheat Penne in Simple Tomato Sauce	Fruit and Nut Trail Mix
W	Baked Egg, Spinach, and Tomato Cups	Waldorf Salad with Perfectly Poached Chicken	Basil and Pine Nut–Topped Sole with Apple Caprese Salad	Fruit and Nut Trail Mix
TH	Baked Egg, Spinach, and Tomato Cups	Waldorf Salad with Perfectly Poached Chicken	Basil and Pine Nut–Topped Sole with Apple Caprese Salad	Fruit and Nut Trail Mix
F	Baked Egg, Spinach, and Tomato Cups	Turkey Meatballs with Whole Wheat Penne in Simple Tomato Sauce	Waldorf Salad with Perfectly Poached Chicken	Fruit and Nut Trail Mix

STEP-BY-STEP PREP:

1. Finely chop the herbs and mince the garlic for all the recipes.

2. Make the tomato sauce for the meatballs (page 187).

3. Preheat the oven to 375°F.

4. Bake the turkey meatballs (page 60), steps 3 and 4.

5. Meanwhile, prep the ingredients, coat a muffin tin with nonstick cooking spray or line with liners, and make the egg mixture for Baked Egg, Spinach, and Tomato Cups (page 55), steps 2 and 3.

6. When the meatballs come out, increase the oven temperature to 400°F. Bake the Egg, Spinach, and Tomato Cups (page 55), step 4.

7. Reduce the oven temperature to 375°F. Line a baking sheet with parchment paper or a silicone baking mat. Bake the Fruit and Nut Trail Mix (page 62), steps 2 and 3. When cool, portion into storage containers.

8. Cook the pasta and assemble with the meatballs and tomato sauce, steps 6 and 7 of the meatball recipe.

9. Poach the chicken for the Waldorf Salad with Perfectly Poached Chicken (page 56), step 1.

10. Meanwhile, prep the vegetables for both the Waldorf salad and the Basil and Pine Nut–Topped Sole with Apple Caprese Salad (page 58).

11. Make the topping and sauté the sole, steps 1 to 3.

12. Make the apple caprese salad and dressing for the sole, steps 4 and 5.

13. Make the dressing and assemble the chicken and salad for the Waldorf salad recipe, steps 2 to 4.

BAKED EGG, SPINACH, AND TOMATO CUPS

Serves 5
Prep time: 15 minutes • **Cook time:** 15 minutes
GLUTEN-FREE • NUT-FREE • VEGETARIAN

Eggs offer the protein needed to keep midmorning hunger pangs at bay. They are also a great grab-and-go option when prepped ahead of time and can be your secret way to serve kids more vegetables. We love this recipe because it incorporates spinach and tomato, helping us get an additional serving of vitamin C, vitamin K, and folate in a great-tasting package.

Nonstick cooking spray
10 large eggs
1 garlic clove, minced
½ tablespoon chopped fresh parsley
½ tablespoon chopped fresh chives

¼ teaspoon freshly ground black pepper
2½ ounces shredded reduced-fat
   Cheddar cheese
2½ cups chopped spinach
1 medium tomato, diced

1. Preheat the oven to 400°F. Coat 10 cups of a muffin tin with cooking spray or line with silicone muffin liners or paper liners.
2. Crack the eggs into a large bowl. Add the garlic, parsley, chives, and pepper and whisk well. Stir in the Cheddar cheese, spinach, and tomato.
3. Divide the egg mixture evenly among the muffin cups, filling about two-thirds full.
4. Bake for about 15 minutes, or until set. Let cool.
5. Place 2 egg cups into each of 5 storage containers.

- **Storage:** Seal and store in the refrigerator for up to 5 days or in the freezer for up to 3 months. To reheat from the freezer, thaw in the refrigerator overnight. Serve cold, or reheat in the microwave for 1 to 2 minutes.

- **Variations:** This recipe is super flexible; if you have a few vegetables left over from a previous meal or a half a block of a different cheese, feel free to swap the ingredients.

   Per Serving: Calories: 232; Total fat: 18g; Carbohydrates: 2g; Fiber: 0.5g; Protein: 17g; Calcium: 203mg; Vitamin D: 84 IU; Potassium: 299mg; Magnesium: 32mg; Sodium: 258mg

WALDORF SALAD WITH PERFECTLY POACHED CHICKEN

Serves 4

Prep time: 15 minutes • **Cook time:** 30 minutes

EGG-FREE • GLUTEN-FREE

Waldorf salad is a classic and a great DASH dish, since it incorporates nuts, fruits, and vegetables. For those who dread vegetables, this may be the perfect option for you. The sweetness of the grapes shines through, and the herbes de Provence—a blend of savory, marjoram, rosemary, thyme, oregano, and lavender—that season the chicken offer a little taste of France. To amp up the flavor, poach the chicken in about 1½ cups of chicken stock with ¼ cup of dry white wine. Add a little whole-grain toast on the side, and you'll have a complete meal.

---

2 (8-ounce) boneless, skinless chicken breasts

2 cups unsalted chicken stock

2 teaspoons herbes de Provence

1 bay leaf

4 cups spinach leaves, stemmed

1 cup seedless grapes, halved

1 medium Gala apple, cut into matchsticks

1 cup chopped celery

¼ cup coarsely chopped walnuts

2 tablespoons crumbled feta cheese

½ cup nonfat plain Greek yogurt

2 tablespoons fresh lemon juice

2 teaspoons honey

¼ teaspoon freshly ground black pepper

1. In a small pot, combine the chicken breasts, chicken stock, herbes de Provence, and bay leaf. If the liquid does not cover the chicken, add a little water. Bring to a boil, then quickly reduce the heat to low, partially cover, and simmer for 5 to 10 minutes, or until the internal temperature of the chicken reaches 165°F. Remove from the heat and let stand in the hot chicken stock for 20 minutes.
2. In a large bowl, combine the spinach, grapes, apple, celery, walnuts, and feta cheese.
3. In a small bowl, whisk together the yogurt, lemon juice, honey, and pepper.
4. Evenly divide the salad among 4 storage containers. Slice the poached chicken and distribute evenly among the containers. Divide the dressing to serve with the salad.

- **Storage:** Seal and store in the refrigerator for up to 5 days. Serve cold.

- **Ingredient tip:** Frozen chicken can help stretch your budget. You can even cook straight from the freezer with a little additional cooking time. To do so, cook the chicken for 50 percent longer, 15 to 20 minutes.

Per Serving: Calories: 295; Total fat: 9g; Carbohydrates: 20g; Fiber: 3g; Protein: 34g; Calcium: 112mg; Vitamin D: 0 IU; Potassium: 643mg; Magnesium: 60mg; Sodium: 557mg

BASIL AND PINE NUT-TOPPED SOLE WITH APPLE CAPRESE SALAD

Serves 3
Prep time: 20 minutes • **Cook time:** 15 minutes
EGG-FREE • GLUTEN-FREE

For this dish, which is a little fancy but full of flavor, we use basil two ways: chopped in the main dish and as a layer in the side salad. Sole is a versatile, mild-flavored fish and has been favored for centuries in French cuisine—especially in the court of Louis XIV. It's great grilled, baked, or pan-seared. Here, sautéed sole serves as a base for a delicious topping of toasted pine nuts, fresh basil, and lemon.

FOR THE SOLE

3 tablespoons pine nuts

3 (4-ounce) sole fillets

½ teaspoon freshly ground black pepper

1 tablespoon extra-virgin olive oil

2 tablespoons fresh lemon juice

2 tablespoons chopped fresh basil

FOR THE SALAD

3 Gala apples, diced

2 tomatoes, diced

3 ounces fresh mozzarella cheese, sliced

6 fresh basil leaves

3 tablespoons balsamic vinegar

3 tablespoons extra-virgin olive oil

Freshly ground black pepper

TO MAKE THE SOLE

1. In a large skillet, toast the pine nuts over medium heat, stirring frequently, for about 3 minutes, or until golden brown. Set aside.
2. Wipe out the skillet. Season the sole with the pepper. Add the oil to the skillet and heat over medium heat. Sauté the fillets for about 2 minutes, or until opaque on the first side. Flip and cook for another 2 minutes. Remove from the skillet and set aside.
3. Pour the lemon juice into the skillet and scrape up any browned bits that remain. Cook the juice for about 1 minute, or until about 1 tablespoon of the juice remains. Add the pine nuts and basil. Remove from the heat.

4. In a large bowl, mix together the apples and tomatoes. Transfer to a low-sided bowl or platter. Place the mozzarella cheese on top. Top the salad with the basil leaves.

5. In a small bowl, whisk together the vinegar and oil. Drizzle on the salad. Sprinkle with pepper to taste.

6. Place a fillet in each of 4 storage containers and top with the sauce. In 4 separate storage containers, evenly divide the caprese salad (without dressing). Store the salad dressing in 2-tablespoon amounts in separate containers.

- **Storage:** Store all the containers in the refrigerator for up to 5 days. Reheat the sole in the oven at 375°F for about 15 minutes. Serve the salad chilled.

- **Variations:** Sole's mild flavor makes it the perfect fit for many different combinations of herbs and vegetables. Don't be afraid to flavor it with dill, thyme, and chives in place of the basil.

Per Serving: Calories: 480; Total fat: 32g; Carbohydrates: 30g; Fiber: 5.5g; Protein: 20g; Calcium: 179mg; Vitamin D: 113 IU; Potassium: 622mg; Magnesium: 56mg; Sodium: 470mg

TURKEY MEATBALLS WITH WHOLE WHEAT PENNE IN SIMPLE TOMATO SAUCE

Serves 4

Prep time: 25 minutes • **Cook time:** 30 minutes

GLUTEN-FREE OPTION (SEE TIP) • VEGETARIAN OPTION (SEE TIP)

Meatballs are always a big hit at the dinner table. They are easy to put together, hold up throughout the week, and are a comfort food for many. For this version, we've gone lean with ground turkey as the base. Our tomato sauce is just a few ingredients and low in sodium and is poured over whole wheat pasta, which offers fiber, protein, B vitamins, and minerals, including magnesium. All this adds up to a better-for-you dish with a lot of nutrition and great flavor.

Simple Tomato Sauce (page 187)

Nonstick cooking spray

1 pound ground turkey

½ cup dried unseasoned bread crumbs

½ cup grated Parmesan cheese

1 tablespoon diced red onion

2 garlic cloves, minced

1 teaspoon chopped fresh basil

¼ cup 1% milk

1 large egg, beaten

8 ounces whole wheat penne pasta

1. Make the tomato sauce. Preheat the oven to 375°F. Coat a sheet pan with cooking spray or line with a silicone baking mat.
2. Bring a large pot of water to a boil for the pasta.
3. In a large bowl, combine the turkey, bread crumbs, Parmesan cheese, onion, garlic, basil, milk, and egg. Mix until well combined. Divide the mixture evenly into 16 portions (smaller than ¼ cup) and roll into meatballs.
4. Place on the prepared sheet pan and bake for 26 to 30 minutes, or until the internal temperature of the meatballs reaches 165°F.
5. Meanwhile, add the pasta to the boiling water and cook until al dente according to the package directions. Drain well in a colander.
6. In a large bowl, toss the pasta with the meatballs and tomato sauce.
7. Divide evenly among 4 storage containers.

- **Storage:** Seal airtight, and store in the refrigerator for up to 5 days. Reheat in the microwave uncovered for 1 to 2 minutes.

- **Gluten-free option:** Spiralized vegetables are a great alternative to whole wheat pasta. Even if you are not looking to avoid gluten, this is a good way to incorporate an extra serving of veggies. A few options include zucchini, carrots, sweet potatoes, and squash. You'll also need to swap in some gluten-free bread crumbs.

- **Vegetarian option:** Make the meatballs with minced white mushrooms in place of ground turkey.

  Per Serving: Calories: 700; Total fat: 33g; Carbohydrates: 74g; Fiber: 8.5g; Protein: 41g; Calcium: 194mg; Vitamin D: 25 IU; Potassium: 447mg; Magnesium: 115mg; Sodium: 532mg

FRUIT AND NUT TRAIL MIX

Serves 5

Prep time: 5 minutes

EGG-FREE • GLUTEN-FREE • DAIRY-FREE OPTION (SEE TIP) • VEGAN OPTION (SEE TIP)

Nuts are a key component of the DASH diet. They provide healthy fats as well as essential vitamins and minerals. When it comes to nuts, portion size is key; it can be easy to overeat. Here, we combine almonds, walnuts, and dark chocolate with dried fruit. Have a portion for a midafternoon snack to give you a much-needed burst of energy to power through the rest of the day.

¼ cup raw almonds

¼ cup walnuts, coarsely chopped

¼ cup maple syrup

¼ cup dried cranberries

¼ cup coarsely chopped dried apricots

¼ cup dark chocolate chips

1. Preheat the oven to 350°F. Line a sheet pan with parchment paper or a silicone baking mat. (Alternatively, you can coat the pan with cooking spray to prevent sticking.)
2. In a medium bowl, combine the almonds, walnuts, maple syrup, cranberries, and apricots. Stir to coat. Spread the mixture out onto the prepared sheet pan.
3. Bake for 20 minutes. Let cool. Add the chocolate chips.
4. Divide evenly among 5 storage containers or plastic bags.

- **Storage:** Store at room temperature for up to 1 month or in the freezer in freezer-safe containers for up to 3 months. Thaw before serving.

- **Variations:** Pistachios and pecans are also possibilities. As for fruit, dried dates, raisins, or pineapples can bring great flavor. Focus on your portion size, select unsalted products, and you can't go wrong.

- **Dairy-free/vegan option:** Use vegan chocolate chips.

Per Serving: Calories: 204; Total fat: 11g; Carbohydrates: 29g; Fiber: 3g; Protein: 3g; Calcium: 48mg; Vitamin D: 0 IU; Potassium: 231mg; Magnesium: 33mg; Sodium: 3mg

Meal Prep 5

For this week's prep, we give you options. The following preps are mostly made with meat, but in the tips, you'll find easy ways to make many of them meatless. Keep in mind that losing the meat doesn't mean losing the protein. Tofu, cheese, nuts, and whole grains are all sources of protein. And remember, protein isn't the only nutrient that keeps hunger at bay; fiber is also important. In the recipes that follow, we've included fiber from whole grains, fruits, and vegetables to keep you feeling full from morning to night.

RECIPE LIST

Arugula and Goat Cheese Pizzas

Chicken and Egg Burritos

Fish Chowder and Crunchy Arugula Salad

Chicken Taco Salad

Energy Snack Bites

SHOPPING LIST

Canned and bottled items

- Beans, black, no-salt-added (1 [15-ounce] can)
- Corn, no-salt-added (1 [15-ounce] can)

Pantry items

- Almond butter (½ cup)
- Almonds, unsalted (¼ cup)
- Black pepper
- Chia seeds (2 tablespoons)
- Chili powder
- Cocoa powder
- Coconut flakes, unsweetened (½ cup)
- Cumin, ground

- Dried thyme
- Flaxseed (2 tablespoons)
- Garlic powder
- Honey
- Nonstick cooking spray
- Oats, rolled (¾ cup)
- Olive oil, extra-virgin
- Onion powder

- Paprika
- Salt

Produce

- Arugula (3 cups)
- Avocados (2)
- Baby spinach (2 cups)
- Carrot (1 large)
- Celery (4 stalks)
- Chives (1 bunch)
- Dill (1 bunch)
- Garlic (1 clove)
- Sunflower seeds (3 tablespoons)
- Vanilla extract
- Lemon (1)
- Lettuce, romaine (1 head)
- Limes (3)
- Pear (1)
- Potatoes (3 medium)
- Onions: red (1 small), yellow (1 small)
- Scallions (1 bunch)
- Tomato (1)

Meat and seafood

- Chicken, ground, lean (1 pound)
- Cod (12 ounces)

Dairy and eggs

- Cheddar cheese, shredded, reduced-fat (2 cups)
- Eggs (6 large)
- Feta cheese (⅓ cup)
- Goat cheese crumbles (5 tablespoons)
- Milk, 1% (8 ounces)
- Yogurt, Greek nonfat plain (6 ounces)

Other

- Tortillas, corn (8) (optional)
- Tortillas, whole wheat, 6-inch (5)
- Tortillas, whole wheat, 10-inch (3)

BE SURE YOU HAVE

- Condiment cups (4)
- Cookie scoop
- Food processor
- Storage containers (10 large)
- Storage containers (3 medium)
- Resealable bags (10)
- Sheet pan (1)
- Toothpicks (optional)

	BREAKFAST	LUNCH	DINNER	SNACK
M	Chicken and Egg Burritos	Fish Chowder and Crunchy Arugula Salad	Chicken Taco Salad	Energy Snack Bites
T	Chicken and Egg Burritos	Chicken Taco Salad	Arugula and Goat Cheese Pizzas	Energy Snack Bites
W	Chicken and Egg Burritos	Arugula and Goat Cheese Pizzas	Fish Chowder and Crunchy Arugula Salad	Energy Snack Bites
TH	Chicken and Egg Burritos	Chicken Taco Salad	Arugula and Goat Cheese Pizzas	Energy Snack Bites
F	Chicken and Egg Burritos	Fish Chowder and Crunchy Arugula Salad	Chicken Taco Salad	Energy Snack Bites

STEP-BY-STEP:

1. Preheat the oven to 400°F. Line a baking sheet with aluminum foil.

2. Chop the vegetables for all of the recipes.

3. Make the topping, and assemble and bake the Arugula and Goat Cheese Pizzas (page 69), steps 2 to 4.

4. Make the Energy Snack Bites (page 71).

5. Make the Fish Chowder and Crunchy Arugula Salad (page 70).

6. Make the Chicken and Egg Burritos (page 66).

7. Make the Greek Yogurt Dill Dressing (page 184) if not using store-bought dressing for the Chicken Taco Salad (page 67).

8. Cook and assemble the Chicken Taco Salad.

CHICKEN AND EGG BURRITOS

Serves 5
Prep time: 5 minutes • **Cook time:** 10 minutes
NUT-FREE • GLUTEN-FREE OPTION (SEE TIP) • VEGETARIAN OPTION (SEE TIP)

As a busy mom, Maria-Paula is always looking for family-friendly breakfast options that can be prepared ahead of time and reheat well. These breakfast burritos are the new favorite of both her daughters and husband because they are hearty and make them feel satisfied until lunchtime. What used to be a meal saved for weekends when time was not an issue has turned into an easy, grab-heat-and-go breakfast for busy mornings.

6 large eggs
2 cups baby spinach
Nonstick cooking spray
8 ounces lean ground chicken
½ teaspoon freshly ground black pepper
½ teaspoon onion powder

½ teaspoon paprika
1 garlic clove, minced
5 (6-inch) whole wheat tortillas
10 tablespoons shredded reduced-fat
    Cheddar cheese

1. In a large bowl, whisk the eggs. Add the spinach and set aside.
2. Coat a large skillet with cooking spray and heat over medium heat. Add the ground chicken, pepper, onion powder, paprika, and garlic and cook, stirring often, until it's no longer pink.
3. Reduce the heat. Add the whisked eggs and continue to cook, stirring often but not constantly, until no liquid egg is visible. Remove from the heat.
4. Evenly distribute the egg and chicken mixture among the tortillas, leaving a 1-inch border around the edges. Sprinkle each with 2 tablespoons of Cheddar cheese. Fold up the bottoms, then the edges, and roll tightly without the contents spilling. Use toothpicks to secure if necessary.

- **Storage:** Store in resealable bags or storage containers in the refrigerator for up to 5 days or in the freezer for up to 1 month. To reheat, wrap in a moist paper towel, and microwave for 45 seconds.

- **Gluten-free option:** Use corn tortillas.

- **Vegetarian option:** Swap the ground chicken with 4 ounces of minced mushrooms.

    Per Serving: Calories: 307; Total fat: 14g; Carbohydrates: 22g; Fiber: 3g; Protein: 25g; Calcium: 236mg; Vitamin D: 51 IU; Potassium: 109mg; Magnesium: 29mg; Sodium: 355mg

CHICKEN TACO SALAD

Serves 4
Prep time: 10 minutes • **Cook time:** 15 minutes
EGG-FREE • GLUTEN-FREE • NUT-FREE • VEGETARIAN OPTION (SEE TIP)

A spin on Taco Tuesday, seasoned chicken can be served in tortillas or on a bed of lettuce (if you'd like to add more leafy greens to the mix) and satisfies even the pickiest eaters. It's also an easy way to incorporate a variety of fresh veggies and herbs into your diet.

Nonstick cooking spray

8 ounces ground chicken

1 (15-ounce) can no-salt-added black beans, drained and rinsed

½ teaspoon ground cumin

½ teaspoon garlic powder

½ teaspoon freshly ground black pepper

¼ teaspoon chili powder

¼ teaspoon paprika

1 (15-ounce) can no-salt-added corn kernels, drained

1 large tomato, diced

¼ cup diced scallions

2 avocados, pitted and cut into chunks

Juice of 2 limes

1 cup packed chopped fresh cilantro leaves

1 head romaine lettuce, coarsely chopped

½ cup shredded reduced-fat Cheddar cheese

½ cup Greek Yogurt Dill Dressing (page 184) or store-bought

8 corn tortillas (optional)

1. Coat a large skillet with cooking spray and heat over medium heat. Add the chicken, beans, cumin, garlic powder, pepper, chili powder, and paprika. Break up the meat and continue stirring until the meat is well cooked and no longer pink. Remove from the heat.
2. In a large bowl, toss together the corn, tomato, scallions, avocados, lime juice, and cilantro.
3. Divide the lettuce among 4 storage containers. Top each with the chicken and bean mixture, then add the corn and vegetable mixture. Sprinkle each with 2 tablespoons of Cheddar cheese. Store the dressing in condiment cups and the tortillas separately (if using).

Continued ❯

- **Storage:** Seal and store in the refrigerator for up to 5 days. No reheating necessary. If you prefer the meat and beans warm, store them separately. To reheat, vent the lid, and microwave for 1 minute.

- **Variation:** For a sweet twist, replace the ground chicken with a 15-ounce can of drained diced mangos or peaches.

- **Vegetarian option:** To make this meal meatless, substitute the ground chicken with another can of beans or 4 ounces of mushrooms.

Per Serving: Calories: 440; Total fat: 23g; Carbohydrates: 38g; Fiber: 15g; Protein: 27g; Calcium: 270mg; Vitamin D: 2 IU; Potassium: 1,131mg; Magnesium: 98mg; Sodium: 182mg

ARUGULA AND GOAT CHEESE PIZZAS

Serves 3
Prep time: 5 minutes • **Cook time:** 10 minutes
NUT-FREE • VEGETARIAN

Who doesn't love it when the weekly menu includes pizza? Especially one that can be put together quickly. The combination of creamy, crunchy, and sweet ingredients in the topping is delightful, and the whole grains in the tortillas mean you won't feel guilty about eating this pizza on the regular.

1 tablespoon extra-virgin olive oil
1 small red onion, thinly sliced
2½ cups arugula, coarsely chopped

3 (10-inch) whole wheat tortillas
1 teaspoon freshly ground black pepper
4½ tablespoons crumbled goat cheese

1. Preheat the oven to 400°F. Line a sheet pan with aluminum foil.
2. In a medium skillet, heat the oil over low heat. Add the onion and cook, stirring occasionally, for about 3 minutes, or until caramelized and light brown. Increase the heat, add the arugula, and cook for a minute or so, or just until wilted. Remove from the heat.
3. Put the tortillas on the prepared sheet pan. Top each tortilla with the caramelized onion and arugula mixture. Sprinkle with the pepper. Top with the goat cheese.
4. Bake for 8 to 10 minutes, or until the tortillas are crisp and the cheese is soft (it won't melt). Let cool for about 5 minutes, then cut each pizza into 4 wedges.

- **Storage:** Store each pizza in a large container or resealable bag for up to 5 days in the refrigerator. Reheat by venting the lid and microwaving for 30 seconds.

Per Serving: Calories: 285; Total fat: 12g; Carbohydrates: 38g; Fiber: 5g; Protein: 8g; Calcium: 43mg; Vitamin D: 0 IU; Potassium: 106mg; Magnesium: 12mg; Sodium: 566mg

FISH CHOWDER AND CRUNCHY ARUGULA SALAD

Serves 3

Prep time: 15 minutes • **Cook time:** 25 minutes

EGG-FREE • GLUTEN-FREE • NUT-FREE

Cod is a great source of protein. It is also flavorful and enriches any meal it accompanies. Pairing it with a crunchy arugula salad creates a combo that gives you a satisfying mix of temperatures and textures.

---

4 tablespoons extra-virgin olive oil, divided

1 small onion, diced

4 celery stalks, diced

2 cups water

2 cups diced potatoes

½ cup sliced carrots

2 teaspoons freshly ground black pepper, divided

2 teaspoons dried thyme

12 ounces cod, cut into ½-inch pieces

1 cup 1% milk

2 tablespoons fresh lemon juice

4½ cups baby arugula

1 pear, diced

⅓ cup crumbled feta cheese

3 tablespoons unsalted roasted sunflower seeds

1. In a large skillet, heat 2 tablespoons of oil over medium heat. Add the onion and celery and sauté for 3 to 4 minutes, or until translucent. Add the water, potatoes, carrots, 1½ teaspoons of pepper, and the thyme and bring to a boil. Reduce the heat, cover, and simmer for about 12 minutes, or until the vegetables are tender.
2. Add the cod and stir. Cook uncovered for 10 minutes. Then add the milk and stir for 1 minute. Remove from the heat and set aside.
3. In a small bowl, combine the lemon juice and the remaining 2 tablespoons of oil and ½ teaspoon of pepper.
4. In a large bowl, mix together the arugula, pear, feta cheese, and sunflower seeds.
5. Divide the chowder, arugula salad, and dressing into separate storage containers.

- **Storage:** Store in the refrigerator for up to 5 days. To reheat the chowder, vent the lid, and microwave for 1 to 2 minutes. Chowder may be frozen for up to 1 month. To reheat from the freezer, thaw in the refrigerator overnight, and reheat as directed for refrigerator.

Per Serving: Calories: 561; Total fat: 26g; Carbohydrates: 45g; Fiber: 8.5g; Protein: 35g; Calcium: 333mg; Vitamin D: 74 IU; Potassium: 1,284mg; Magnesium: 139mg; Sodium: 536mg

ENERGY SNACK BITES

Serves 5
Prep time: 10 minutes, plus 20 minutes to firm up
DAIRY-FREE • EGG-FREE • VEGETARIAN • GLUTEN-FREE OPTION (SEE TIP) •
NUT-FREE OPTION (SEE TIP)

As on-the-go moms, both Katie and Maria-Paula love these easy-to-prep, nutty but sweet snacks. Everyone loves eating them, but we also love that they store well and can be ready for a surprise playdate or an extra practice. As a runner, Maria-Paula also uses them to fuel her runs.

¾ cup rolled oats, plus more as needed

½ cup unsweetened coconut flakes

¼ cup chopped raw almonds

2 tablespoons unsweetened cocoa powder

2 tablespoons flaxseed

2 tablespoons chia seeds

½ cup almond butter, plus more as needed

⅓ cup honey

1 teaspoon vanilla extract

¼ teaspoon salt

1. In a large bowl, combine the oats, coconut flakes, almonds, cocoa, flaxseed, chia seeds, almond butter, honey, vanilla, and salt. Stir until all ingredients are well combined. The goal is to achieve a sticky dough that can be formed into balls and will hold together. For a mixture that is too dry, add more almond butter. For a mixture that is too wet, add more oats.
2. Refrigerate the mixture for about 20 minutes to firm it up so you form the balls more easily.
3. Using a cookie scoop to help you keep them uniform, form into 15 balls about 1 inch in diameter.
4. Place 3 bites in each of 5 resealable bags.

- **Storage:** Store in the refrigerator for up to 2 weeks or in the freezer for up to 3 months.

- **Gluten-free option:** Use certified gluten-free oats.

- **Nut-free option:** Use sunflower seed butter instead of almond butter, and sunflower seeds in place of almonds.

  Per Serving (3 bites): Calories: 398; Total fat: 26g; Carbohydrates: 39g; Fiber: 9g; Protein: 11g; Calcium: 155mg; Vitamin D: 0 IU; Potassium: 382mg; Magnesium: 134mg; Sodium: 179mg

Meal Prep 6

This week, we share a few of our favorite ways to save time, incorporate more healthy-for-you DASH superstars, and keep you satisfied. The recipe count is now up to six: We've added a second breakfast option for a little more variety. Finally, we thought about recipes with opportunities for creative tweaking. That way, if you ever plan to repeat this meal prep week, you can make the recipes seem brand new simply by swapping out a few of the main components. Think chicken instead of tuna, or peaches for apples when they're in season. Add berries in the summer. Incorporating seasonal fruits and vegetables is a great way to keep your recipes evolving. DASH, after all, isn't a diet; it's a heart-healthy lifestyle.

RECIPE LIST

Apple-Cinnamon Overnight Oats

Great Greens Smoothie Bowl

Mediterranean Pasta Salad

Tuna Kebabs with Fresh Vegetables and Cilantro Rice

Turkey Burgers with Roasted Carrots and Beets

Fresh Fruit with Peanut Butter Yogurt Dip

SHOPPING LIST

Canned and bottled items

- Olives, Kalamata (½ cup)

Pantry items

- Black pepper
- Cinnamon, ground
- Coconut flakes, unsweetened (¼ cup)
- Dried basil
- Dried oregano

- Hamburger buns, whole wheat (4)
- Honey
- Mustard, whole-grain
- Nonstick cooking spray
- Nutmeg, ground

- Oats, rolled (1½ cups)
- Olive oil, extra-virgin
- Pasta, penne, whole wheat (6 ounces)
- Peanut butter (½ cup)
- Red pepper flakes (optional)
- Rice, brown (1 cup)
- Salt
- Sugar, brown (3 tablespoons)
- Vinegar, balsamic
- Walnuts, chopped (3 tablespoons)

Produce

- Apples: Gala (4 medium), green (1 medium)
- Baby spinach (4 cups)
- Banana (1)
- Beets (4)
- Bell pepper, green (1)
- Carrots (8)
- Cilantro (1 bunch)
- Garlic (4 cloves)
- Kale (2 cups)
- Lemons (2)
- Limes (1)
- Mushrooms, cremini (8)
- Onions, red (2 medium)
- Orange (1 medium)
- Parsley (¼ bunch)
- Strawberries (1 pint)
- Tomato (1 medium)
- Tomatoes, grape (1 pint)

Frozen foods

- Mango chunks (1 cup)

Meat and seafood

- Tuna steaks (12 ounces)
- Turkey, ground (1 pound)

Dairy and eggs

- Cheddar cheese (4 ounces)
- Milk, 1% (2½ cups)
- Parmesan cheese, grated (3 tablespoons)
- Yogurt, Greek nonfat plain (½ cup)

BE SURE YOU HAVE

- Bamboo skewers (4)
- Blender
- Condiment cups (5)
- Grill (optional)
- Mason jars (3)
- Resealable bag (1)

- Sheet pan (1)
- Storage containers (8 large)
- Storage containers (4 large, divided)
- Storage containers (9 medium)
- Storage containers (5 small)
- Zester or grater

	BREAKFAST	LUNCH	DINNER	SNACK
M	Apple-Cinnamon Overnight Oats	Mediterranean Pasta Salad	Turkey Burgers with Roasted Carrots and Beets	Fresh Fruit with Peanut Butter Yogurt Dip
T	Great Greens Smoothie Bowl	Tuna Kebabs with Fresh Vegetables and Cilantro Rice	Mediterranean Pasta Salad	Fresh Fruit with Peanut Butter Yogurt Dip
W	Apple-Cinnamon Overnight Oats	Turkey Burgers with Roasted Carrots and Beets	Tuna Kebabs with Fresh Vegetables and Cilantro Rice	Fresh Fruit with Peanut Butter Yogurt Dip
TH	Great Greens Smoothie Bowl	Turkey Burgers with Roasted Carrots and Beets	Tuna Kebabs with Fresh Vegetables and Cilantro Rice	Fresh Fruit with Peanut Butter Yogurt Dip
F	Apple-Cinnamon Overnight Oats	Mediterranean Pasta Salad	Turkey Burgers with Roasted Carrots and Beets	Fresh Fruit with Peanut Butter Yogurt Dip

STEP-BY-STEP PREP:

1. Chop any fresh herbs and mince the garlic for all recipes.

2. Preheat the oven to 375°F.

3. Prep and roast the carrots and beets (page 105) for the turkey burgers.

4. Marinate the tuna for the Tuna Kebabs with Fresh Vegetables and Cilantro Rice (page 79), step 1.

5. Make the Cilantro Rice (page 108) for the tuna kebabs.

6. Preheat the grill (or stove) and soak the bamboo skewers for the tuna kebabs.

7. Prepare the vegetables for the kebabs, Mediterranean Pasta Salad (page 78), and turkey burgers (page 81).

8. Make and assemble the pasta salad.

9. Thread the skewers and cook the tuna kebabs (page 79), steps 5 and 6.

10. Cook the turkey burgers and assemble them (page 81), steps 2 to 5.

11. Prep the ingredients, assemble, and store the Apple-Cinnamon Overnight Oats (page 76), Great Greens Smoothie Bowl (page 77), and Fresh Fruit with Peanut Butter Yogurt Dip (page 83).

APPLE-CINNAMON OVERNIGHT OATS

Serves 3
Prep time: 15 minutes, plus overnight to soak
EGG-FREE • VEGETARIAN • GLUTEN-FREE OPTION (SEE TIP)

Overnight oats are a perfect solution for busy mornings. Prep, store, and add a little milk the night before you plan to eat them for a breakfast that is nutritious and filling. Katie likes to top her overnight oats with fresh fruit, which means a little preparation to keep those apples from browning: Add 2 tablespoons of honey to some water, and soak the apples for 30 seconds to prevent browning and add a little sweetness.

---

2 medium Gala apples, diced
1½ cups rolled oats
3 tablespoons coarsely chopped walnuts
3 tablespoons brown sugar

1½ tablespoons ground cinnamon
Pinch ground nutmeg
1½ cups 1% milk

1. Put the diced apples in a storage container.
2. In a large bowl, mix the oats, walnuts, brown sugar, cinnamon, and nutmeg. Divide evenly among 3 mason jars and seal the jars.
3. The evening before you plan to have this for breakfast, add ½ cup of milk to each jar of oat mixture and let sit in the refrigerator overnight.
4. In the morning, top each with ½ cup of diced apples.

- **Storage:** Store the jars of dry ingredients at room temperature for 1 to 2 weeks. Store the diced apples in the refrigerator for up to 5 days.

- **Variations:** Ditch the fresh fruits and raid your pantry for dried fruit. Dried apricots, cranberries, and raisins are all great ingredients when it comes to overnight oats. Use about 2 tablespoons per serving.

- **Gluten-free option:** Use certified gluten-free oats.

  Per Serving: Calories: 368; Total fat: 9g; Carbohydrates: 66g; Fiber: 9g; Protein: 11g; Calcium: 228mg; Vitamin D: 50 IU; Potassium: 331mg; Magnesium: 55mg; Sodium: 69mg

GREAT GREENS SMOOTHIE BOWL

Serves 2
Prep time: 10 minutes • **Cook time:** 3 minutes
EGG-FREE • GLUTEN-FREE • NUT-FREE • VEGETARIAN

Smoothie bowls have exploded in popularity lately, and for good reason—they're healthy, fast, and fun. They are a great way to add a few servings of fruits and vegetables to your morning. When you top them off, consider foods that offer a little additional color and texture. Your goal is to make them pop. They are also a great creative outlet for kids. And when you finish posting your photos on social media, they're an art project you can eat.

¼ cup unsweetened coconut flakes

1 green apple, thinly sliced, divided

1 banana, cut into chunks

1 cup frozen mango chunks

1 cup chopped kale leaves

1 cup baby spinach

1 cup 1% milk

½ lemon, thinly sliced

1. In a small dry skillet, toast the coconut flakes over medium heat for 2 to 3 minutes, or until lightly browned. Set side.
2. In a blender, combine three-quarters of the apple slices, all the banana, mango, kale, spinach, and milk and blend until well combined. Pour into a storage container. Store the smoothie, remaining apple slices, the lemon slices, and toasted coconut separately.
3. For each serving, pour half the smoothie into a bowl. Top with half the remaining apple slices, half the lemon slices, and coconut flakes.

• **Storage:** Store in the refrigerator for up to 5 days, or freeze for up to 3 months in freezer-safe containers. To thaw, refrigerate overnight.

• **Variations:** Smoothies are a great place to easily add protein. Consider adding ½ cup of Greek yogurt or a scoop of whey protein to your morning bowl. You'll feel full longer.

Per Serving: Calories: 262; Total fat: 6.5g; Carbohydrates: 47g; Fiber: 7.5g; Protein: 8g; Calcium: 196mg; Vitamin D: 50 IU; Potassium: 351mg; Magnesium: 44mg; Sodium: 94mg

MEDITERRANEAN PASTA SALAD

Serves 3
Prep time: 10 minutes • **Cook time:** 15 minutes
EGG-FREE • NUT-FREE • VEGETARIAN • GLUTEN-FREE OPTION (SEE TIP)

The Mediterranean and DASH diets are similar, with lots of fruits and vegetables, whole grains, seafood, nuts, seeds, and olive oil. Here, we combine the benefits of both. In this recipe, you'll find heart-healthy fats from the olives and olive oil. The whole wheat pasta provides fiber and essential nutrients.

6 ounces whole wheat penne pasta

2 tablespoons extra-virgin olive oil

2 garlic cloves, minced

2 teaspoons dried oregano

1 teaspoon dried basil

3 cups spinach leaves, stemmed

1 tablespoon balsamic vinegar

1 pint grape tomatoes, halved

½ cup pitted Kalamata olives, sliced

3 tablespoons grated Parmesan cheese

¼ teaspoon red pepper flakes (optional)

1. Bring a large pot of water to a boil. Add the pasta and cook until al dente according to the package directions. Drain well.
2. In a large skillet, heat the oil over medium heat. Add the garlic and cook, stirring constantly, for 30 seconds to 1 minute, or until fragrant. Add the oregano, basil, and spinach and sauté for about 3 minutes, or until the spinach is fully cooked. Remove from the heat and stir in the vinegar.
3. In a large bowl, combine the pasta, spinach mixture, tomatoes, and olives. Top with the Parmesan cheese and red pepper flakes (if using).
4. Divide evenly among 3 storage containers.

- **Storage:** Store in the refrigerator for up to 5 days or in the freezer for up to 3 months. To thaw, refrigerate overnight. This dish can be served hot or cold. Although it will reheat nicely, reheating isn't necessary. If desired, reheat in the microwave for 1 to 2 minutes or over medium heat on the stovetop until warm.

- **Gluten-free option:** Use gluten-free penne.

  Per Serving: Calories: 435; Total fat: 20g; Carbohydrates: 61g; Fiber: 8.5g; Protein: 13g; Calcium: 110mg; Vitamin D: 1 IU; Potassium: 343mg; Magnesium: 110mg; Sodium: 546mg

TUNA KEBABS WITH FRESH VEGETABLES AND CILANTRO RICE

Serves 3
Prep time: 20 minutes, plus 30 minutes to marinate • **Cook time:** 20 minutes
DAIRY-FREE • EGG-FREE • GLUTEN-FREE • NUT-FREE

Fresh tuna makes for a nice twist on the typical grilled kebab. It's a hearty enough fish to take a marinade and sturdy enough to hold together on a skewer. We've added a few vegetables that are also enhanced by the heat: red onion, green bell pepper, and cremini mushrooms. Pairing the kebab with a brown rice side dish provides additional nutrients, including fiber, B vitamins, magnesium, phosphorus, and calcium.

Juice of 1 orange

Juice of 1 lemon

Juice of 1 lime

2 garlic cloves, minced

1 tablespoon honey

¼ cup extra-virgin olive oil,
   plus 2 teaspoons (if not grilling)

¼ teaspoon freshly ground black pepper

12 ounces tuna, cut into 2-inch chunks

1½ cups Cilantro Rice (page 108)

Nonstick cooking spray

1 medium red onion, cut into 2-inch chunks

1 green bell pepper, cut into 2-inch chunks

8 small cremini mushrooms

1. In a small bowl, whisk together the orange juice, lemon juice, lime juice, garlic, honey, ¼ cup of oil, and the black pepper. Pour into a large resealable bag and add the tuna. Marinate for 30 minutes or up to 24 hours.
2. Make the cilantro rice.
3. If grilling, soak the bamboo skewers in water for at least 30 minutes before cooking.
4. Coat the grill grates with cooking spray. Preheat the grill to medium-high heat. (Alternatively, heat 2 teaspoons of oil in a skillet over medium-high heat.)
5. Thread the tuna, onion, bell pepper, and mushrooms onto the bamboo skewers, alternating the ingredients.

Continued ❯

6. Grill for 4 minutes on each side for medium-rare, or add a few minutes if medium is desired. (If cooking in a skillet, sauté for 8 to 10 minutes, or until the tuna is browned, 8 to 10 minutes.)
7. Divide the kebabs and rice into 3 divided containers.

- **Storage:** Store in the refrigerator for up to 5 days or in the freezer for up to 3 months. To thaw, refrigerate overnight. Reheat the kebab wrapped in foil in a 350°F oven for 30 minutes. Add a tablespoon of water to the rice, and reheat uncovered in the microwave for 1 to 2 minutes.

Per Serving: Calories: 387; Total fat: 14g; Carbohydrates: 39g; Fiber: 3g; Protein: 31g; Calcium: 38mg; Vitamin D: 73 IU; Potassium: 979mg; Magnesium: 90mg; Sodium: 332mg

TURKEY BURGERS WITH ROASTED CARROTS AND BEETS

Serves 4
Prep time: 10 minutes • **Cook time:** 10 minutes
EGG-FREE • NUT-FREE

This turkey burger is the perfect choice when you're craving something hearty. To achieve this, we've topped a grilled turkey patty with Cheddar cheese, chopped kale, tomato, and onion, all enhanced with a little whole-grain mustard. To help you get your vegetable servings, we've paired the burgers with a roasted carrot and beet side salad.

Roasted Carrots and Beets (page 105)

Nonstick cooking spray

2 tablespoons extra-virgin olive oil (if not grilling)

1 pound ground turkey

¼ teaspoon salt

¼ teaspoon freshly ground black pepper

4 (1-ounce) Cheddar cheese slices

4 whole wheat hamburger buns

2 tablespoons whole-grain mustard

1 cup chopped kale leaves

1 medium tomato, sliced

½ medium red onion, sliced

1. Roast the carrots and beets. Coat the grill grates with cooking spray. Preheat the grill to high heat. (Alternatively, heat the oil in a skillet over medium-high heat.)
2. Form the turkey into 4 equal patties and season with the salt and pepper. Grill the patties covered for 5 minutes. Flip and continue to cook covered for an additional 5 minutes. (Same time if cooking in a skillet.)
3. Place a patty and a slice of Cheddar cheese in each of 4 storage containers. Store the buns, mustard, kale, tomato, onion, and roasted carrots, and beets separately.

Continued ❯

4. When ready to serve, reheat the patties for 1 minute. Top with the cheese and heat together long enough for the cheese to melt. Split and toast the buns. Spread the toasted buns with the mustard and assemble the burgers with the kale, tomato, and onion.

5. Serve with the roasted vegetables.

- **Storage:** Store in the refrigerator for up to 5 days.

- **Variations:** No whole-grain mustard at home? Top with ketchup, mayonnaise, or sliced avocado instead.

  Per Serving: Calories: 690; Total fat: 41g; Carbohydrates: 46g; Fiber: 9.5g; Protein: 32g; Calcium: 398mg; Vitamin D: 6 IU; Potassium: 1,033mg; Magnesium: 120mg; Sodium: 910mg

FRESH FRUIT WITH PEANUT BUTTER YOGURT DIP

Serves 5
Prep time: 10 minutes
EGG-FREE • GLUTEN-FREE • VEGETARIAN

This is the perfect pick-me-up for long afternoons at the office or at school. With all the macronutrients—proteins, carbohydrates, and fat—this snack will leave you full and energized to finish the day. Greek yogurt makes a great creamy base for all types of dips, both savory and sweet. Here, we used peanut butter, which is basically savory, but then gave it a touch of sweetness with cinnamon and nutmeg.

½ cup nonfat plain Greek yogurt
½ cup peanut butter
¼ teaspoon ground cinnamon

Pinch ground nutmeg
2 medium Gala apples, sliced
1 cup whole strawberries

1. In a small bowl, whisk together the yogurt, peanut butter, cinnamon, and nutmeg. Serve with the apple slices.
2. Divide the apples and strawberries, and dip evenly among 5 storage containers.

- **Storage:** Seal and store in the refrigerator for up to 5 days. The dip can be frozen for up to 3 months in freezer-safe containers. To thaw, refrigerate overnight.

- **Variations:** Unsalted pretzel sticks or dried fruit chips can offer a little crunch to the mix. Or try the Super-Simple Granola (page 91) for a crunchy topping.

Per Serving: Calories: 209; Total fat: 13g; Carbohydrates: 18g; Fiber: 3.5g; Protein: 8g; Calcium: 45mg; Vitamin D: 0 IU; Potassium: 290mg; Magnesium: 50mg; Sodium: 118mg

Pineapple and Shrimp Skewers
Page 149

PART THREE

MORE MEAL PREP RECIPES PLUS DASH STAPLES

In this section, you'll find a variety of DASH-friendly recipes that you can swap into the previous meal preps when you're ready for a change or want to add an extra recipe or two during the week. We've included breakfast, lunch, and dinner options, plus a good selection of soups, salads, side dishes, and sauces. For entrées, there are meat, seafood, and poultry dishes as well as vegetarian dishes—great recipes for you to invent a different meal prep each week. Our focus was very much on flavor, but also on "nutrition by addition," which means including generous portions of filling and nutrient-rich foods. We want you to embrace those good-for-you foods from DASH and realize that adding an extra serving of vegetables or including a serving of whole grains goes a long way in getting you more essential nutrients that support heart health.

Blueberry Waffles
Page 88

CHAPTER 3

Breakfast

BLUEBERRY WAFFLES

Makes 8 waffles
Prep time: 5 minutes • **Cook time:** 15 minutes
VEGETARIAN • GLUTEN-FREE OPTION (SEE TIP)

Whole grains are the best way to start the day because meals higher in fiber keep you satisfied longer. These waffles get their sweetness from a little sugar and a lot of fruit. They're topped with store-bought maple almond butter—Maria-Paula's favorite sweet and savory blend.

2 cups whole wheat flour

1 tablespoon baking powder

1 teaspoon ground cinnamon

2 tablespoons sugar

2 large eggs

3 tablespoons unsalted butter, melted

3 tablespoons nonfat plain Greek yogurt

1½ cups 1% milk

2 teaspoons vanilla extract

4 ounces blueberries

Nonstick cooking spray

½ cup maple almond butter

1. Preheat a waffle iron.
2. In a large bowl, stir together the flour, baking powder, cinnamon, and sugar.
3. In a small bowl, whisk together the eggs, melted butter, yogurt, milk, and vanilla. Combine well.
4. Add the wet ingredients to the dry mix and whisk until well combined. Do not over whisk; it's okay if the mixture has some lumps. Fold in the blueberries.
5. Coat the waffle iron with cooking spray. Ladle ⅓ cup of the batter onto the iron and cook until the waffles are lightly browned and slightly crisp. Repeat with the rest of the batter.
6. Place 2 waffles in each of 4 storage containers. Store the almond butter in 4 condiment cups. To serve, top each warm waffle with 1 tablespoon of maple almond butter.

- **Storage:** Store in the refrigerator for up to 4 days. To reheat, put a waffle in the toaster for 1 to 1½ minutes. To freeze, place parchment paper between the waffles, and store for up to 3 months. To reheat, put in the toaster for 2 to 3 minutes.

- **Substitution tip:** Use your favorite nut butter instead of maple almond. You can also use frozen blueberries in place of fresh.

- **Variations:** Sprinkle with 1 teaspoon of powdered sugar, or pair with vanilla Greek yogurt for a delicious and satisfying combination.

- **Gluten-free option:** Use an all-purpose gluten-free flour.

  Per Serving (2 waffles): Calories: 647; Total fat: 37g; Carbohydrates: 67g; Fiber: 9.5g; Protein: 22g; Calcium: 250mg; Vitamin D: 58 IU; Potassium: 296mg; Magnesium: 89mg; Sodium: 156mg

APPLE PANCAKES

Makes 16 pancakes
Prep time: 5 minutes • **Cook time:** 5 minutes
VEGETARIAN • EGG-FREE OPTION (SEE TIP)

The DASH diet is about small enhancements to foods you already eat. These pancakes contain fiber due to the whole wheat flour. The apple adds a little natural sugar, and cinnamon provides a warm aroma and a nice complement to that sweetness. Pair the dish with a few chopped walnuts for some healthy fats and to get some vitamin E, calcium, magnesium, potassium, iron, and zinc.

¼ cup extra-virgin olive oil, divided

1 cup whole wheat flour

2 teaspoons baking powder

1 teaspoon baking soda

1 teaspoon ground cinnamon

1 cup 1% milk

2 large eggs

1 medium Gala apple, diced

2 tablespoons maple syrup

¼ cup chopped walnuts

1. Set aside 1 teaspoon of oil to use for oiling a griddle or skillet. In a large bowl, stir together the flour, baking powder, baking soda, cinnamon, milk, eggs, apple, and the remaining oil.
2. Heat a griddle or skillet over medium-high heat and coat with the reserved oil. Working in batches, pour in about ¼ cup of the batter for each pancake. Cook until browned on both sides.
3. Place 4 pancakes into each of 4 medium storage containers and the maple syrup in 4 small containers. To serve, sprinkle each serving with 1 tablespoon of walnuts and drizzle with ½ tablespoon of maple syrup.

- **Storage:** Store in the refrigerator for up to 5 days or in the freezer for up to 1 month. Reheat in the microwave for 30 seconds to 1 minute. If reheating from frozen, microwave wrapped in a wet paper towel for 90 seconds to 2 minutes.

- **Egg-free option:** Swap in ¼ cup of unsweetened applesauce for the eggs.

Per Serving (4 pancakes): Calories: 378; Total fat: 22g; Carbohydrates: 39g; Fiber: 5g; Protein: 10g; Calcium: 124mg; Vitamin D: 50 IU; Potassium: 334mg; Magnesium: 65mg; Sodium: 65mg

SUPER-SIMPLE GRANOLA

Serves 8
Prep time: 10 minutes • **Cook time:** 25 minutes
DAIRY-FREE • EGG-FREE • VEGETARIAN • GLUTEN-FREE OPTION (SEE TIP) • VEGAN OPTION (SEE TIP)

Don't be intimidated by homemade granola—it's relatively quick and easy to make. Plus, making granola from scratch is a great way to save a little money and control the salt and sugar in your food. It's also a versatile ingredient to add to yogurt, oatmeal, and fruit salads. Additionally, you can use this as the breading for Breaded and Baked Chicken Tenders (page 166) or to top an apple pie.

¼ cup extra-virgin olive oil

¼ cup honey

½ teaspoon ground cinnamon

½ teaspoon vanilla extract

¼ teaspoon salt

2 cups rolled oats

½ cup chopped walnuts

½ cup slivered almonds

1. Preheat the oven to 350°F. Line a sheet pan with parchment paper or a silicone baking mat. (Alternatively, you can coat the pan with cooking spray to prevent sticking.)
2. In a large bowl, whisk together the oil, honey, cinnamon, vanilla, and salt. Add the oats, walnuts, and almonds. Stir to coat. Spread the mixture out onto the prepared sheet pan.
3. Bake for 20 minutes. Let cool.

- **Storage:** Divide into 8 storage containers, and store at room temperature for up to 1 month or in the freezer for up to 3 months. Thaw before serving.

- **Gluten-free option:** Use certified gluten-free oats.

- **Vegan option:** Use maple syrup instead of honey.

  Per Serving: Calories: 254; Total fat: 16g; Carbohydrates: 25g; Fiber: 3.5g; Protein: 5g; Calcium: 38mg; Vitamin D: 0 IU; Potassium: 163mg; Magnesium: 50mg; Sodium: 73mg

SAVORY YOGURT BOWLS

Serves 4

Prep time: 15 minutes

EGG-FREE • GLUTEN-FREE • VEGETARIAN

Many people think of a morning parfait as something sweet, but Greek yogurt provides a creamy, versatile base for great savory creations. Shake things up and reach for a few different flavors to add to your yogurt, such as beets, avocado, and mint or roasted carrots and sweet potatoes paired with parsley and thyme. This bowl is also a clever way to get a few more servings of vegetables.

1 medium cucumber, diced

½ cup pitted Kalamata olives, halved

2 tablespoons fresh lemon juice

1 tablespoon extra-virgin olive oil

1 teaspoon dried oregano

¼ teaspoon freshly ground black pepper

2 cups nonfat plain Greek yogurt

½ cup slivered almonds

1. In a small bowl, mix together the cucumber, olives, lemon juice, oil, oregano, and pepper.
2. Divide the yogurt evenly among 4 storage containers. Top with the cucumber-olive mix and almonds.

- **Storage:** Seal and store for up to 5 days in the refrigerator.
- **Ingredient tip:** Add any leftover cooked veggies you might have to this yogurt bowl. It helps your wallet and reduces food waste. It will also save you a little prep time.

Per Serving: Calories: 240; Total fat: 16g; Carbohydrates: 10g; Fiber: 2g; Protein: 16g; Calcium: 183mg; Vitamin D: 0 IU; Potassium: 353mg; Magnesium: 57mg; Sodium: 350mg

ENERGY SUNRISE MUFFINS

Makes 16 muffins
Prep time: 15 minutes • **Cook time:** 25 minutes
DAIRY-FREE • VEGETARIAN • GLUTEN-FREE OPTION (SEE TIP)

Sweet and hearty, the combination of orange and honey and the textures of shredded apple and carrots give these grab-and-go muffins a special place in Maria-Paula's and her girls' weekday mornings. They are a great source of fiber, which aids in digestion, as well as beta-carotene (vitamin A) and vitamin C, two powerful antioxidants.

Nonstick cooking spray
2 cups whole wheat flour
2 teaspoons baking soda
2 teaspoons ground cinnamon
1 teaspoon ground ginger
¼ teaspoon salt
3 large eggs
½ cup packed brown sugar
⅓ cup unsweetened applesauce
¼ cup honey

¼ cup vegetable or canola oil
1 teaspoon grated orange zest
Juice of 1 medium orange
2 teaspoons vanilla extract
2 cups shredded carrots
1 large apple, peeled and grated
½ cup golden raisins
½ cup chopped pecans
½ cup unsweetened coconut flakes

1. If you can fit two 12-cup muffin tins side by side in your oven, then leave a rack in the middle. Otherwise, position racks in the upper and lower thirds of the oven and preheat the oven to 350°F.
2. Coat 16 cups of the muffin tins with cooking spray or line with paper liners.
3. In a large bowl, combine the flour, baking soda, cinnamon, ginger, and salt. Set aside.
4. In a medium bowl, whisk together the eggs, brown sugar, applesauce, honey, oil, orange zest, orange juice, and vanilla until combined. Add the carrots and apple and whisk again.
5. Mix the dry and wet ingredients together with a spatula. Fold in the raisins, pecans, and coconut. Mix everything together once again, just until well combined.
6. Spoon the batter into the muffin cups, filling them to the top.

Continued ❯

7. Bake for 20 to 25 minutes, or until a wooden toothpick inserted into the middle of the center muffin comes out clean (switching racks halfway through if baking on 2 racks).
8. Cool for 5 minutes in the tins, then transfer to a wire rack to cool for an additional 5 minutes. Cool completely before storing in containers.

- **Storage:** Cover leftover muffins, and store at room temperature for 2 days or in the refrigerator for 1 week. May freeze up to 1 month and thaw in the refrigerator overnight before serving.

- **Gluten-free option:** Use all-purpose gluten-free flour.

  Per Serving (1 muffin): Calories: 292; Total fat: 14g; Carbohydrates: 42g; Fiber: 4.5g; Protein: 5g; Calcium: 41mg; Vitamin D: 10 IU; Potassium: 274mg; Magnesium: 42mg; Sodium: 84mg

SPINACH, EGG, AND CHEESE BREAKFAST QUESADILLAS

Serves 4
Prep time: 10 minutes • **Cook time:** 15 minutes
NUT-FREE • VEGETARIAN • GLUTEN-FREE OPTION (SEE TIP)

Breakfast quesadillas are a simple and satisfying start to your day. The protein from the eggs and cheese combined with the fiber in the whole wheat tortillas work together to keep you fuller longer, helping you get through any midmorning cravings. Spinach is packed with potassium, calcium, and beta-carotene (vitamin A), all nutrients that benefit your heart health.

1½ tablespoons extra-virgin olive oil
½ medium onion, diced
1 medium red bell pepper, diced
4 large eggs
⅛ teaspoon salt
⅛ teaspoon freshly ground black pepper

4 cups baby spinach
½ cup crumbled feta cheese
Nonstick cooking spray
4 (6-inch) whole wheat tortillas, divided
1 cup shredded part-skim low-moisture
   mozzarella cheese, divided

1. In a large skillet, heat the oil over medium heat. Add the onion and bell pepper and sauté for about 5 minutes, or until soft.
2. In a medium bowl, whisk together the eggs, salt, and black pepper. Stir in the spinach and feta cheese. Add the egg mixture to the skillet and scramble for about 2 minutes, or until the eggs are cooked. Remove from the heat.
3. Coat a clean skillet with cooking spray and add 2 tortillas. Place one-quarter of the spinach-egg mixture on one side of each tortilla. Sprinkle each with ¼ cup of mozzarella cheese. Fold the other halves of the tortillas down to close the quesadillas and brown for about 1 minute. Flip and cook for another minute on the other side. Repeat with the remaining 2 tortillas and ½ cup of mozzarella cheese.
4. Cut each quesadilla in half or wedges. Divide among 4 storage containers or reusable bags.

Continued ❯

SPINACH, EGG, AND CHEESE BREAKFAST QUESADILLAS *Continued*

- **Storage:** Store in the refrigerator for up to 4 days or in the freezer for up to 3 months. When reheating, coat a small skillet with cooking spray, and reheat the quesadilla over medium heat for 1 to 2 minutes. Or reheat in the microwave for 1 minute. If reheating from frozen, microwave on medium for 2 minutes, place in a small skillet coated with cooking spray, and heat over medium heat for 1 to 2 minutes.

- **Substitution tip:** You can use frozen instead of fresh spinach. You'll need 2 ounces of frozen spinach that has been thawed, drained, and squeezed of its moisture.

- **Gluten-free option:** Use corn tortillas.

  Per Serving: Calories: 453; Total fat: 28g; Carbohydrates: 28g; Fiber: 4.5g; Protein: 23g; Calcium: 394mg; Vitamin D: 45 IU; Potassium: 205mg; Magnesium: 59mg; Sodium: 837mg

SIMPLE CHEESE AND BROCCOLI OMELETS

Serves 4

Prep time: 5 minutes • **Cook time:** 10 minutes

GLUTEN-FREE • NUT-FREE • VEGETARIAN

Omelets that combine eggs, cheese, and vegetables give you a nice balance of high-quality protein, fiber, and DASH minerals—calcium, potassium, and magnesium. Here, broccoli is providing the magnesium, but you can easily swap it out for spinach, cauliflower, or potatoes and still get that boost.

---

3 tablespoons extra-virgin olive oil, divided

2 cups chopped broccoli

8 large eggs

¼ cup 1% milk

½ teaspoon freshly ground black pepper

8 tablespoons shredded reduced-fat Monterey Jack cheese, divided

1. In a nonstick skillet, heat 1 tablespoon of oil over medium-high heat. Add the broccoli and sauté, stirring occasionally, for 3 to 5 minutes, or until the broccoli turns bright green. Scrape into a bowl.
2. In a small bowl, beat together the eggs, milk, and pepper.
3. Wipe out the skillet and heat ½ tablespoon of oil. Add one-quarter of the egg mixture and tilt the skillet to ensure an even layer. Cook for 2 minutes and then add 2 tablespoons of cheese and one-quarter of the broccoli. Use a spatula to fold into an omelet.
4. Repeat step 3 with the remaining 1½ tablespoons of oil, remaining egg mixture, 6 tablespoons of cheese, and remaining broccoli to make a total of 4 omelets. Divide into 4 storage containers.

- **Storage:** Store in the refrigerator for up to 5 days. To reheat, microwave for 30 seconds to 1 minute, bake at 325°F for up to 10 minutes, or heat in a skillet with a little bit of olive oil until warm.

- **Variations:** Swap in almost any veggie for the broccoli: Mushrooms, tomatoes, cauliflower, and bell peppers are all great options.

  Per Serving: Calories: 292; Total fat: 23g; Carbohydrates: 4g; Fiber: 1g; Protein: 18g; Calcium: 199mg; Vitamin D: 89 IU; Potassium: 308mg; Magnesium: 25mg; Sodium: 282mg

CREAMY AVOCADO AND EGG SALAD SANDWICHES

Serves 4
Prep time: 5 minutes • **Cook time:** 15 minutes
NUT-FREE • VEGETARIAN

Avocado gives these classic egg salad sandwiches an interesting and nutritious twist. Rich in potassium, heart-healthy monounsaturated fats, and fiber, avocados are a great nutritious staple to add to your DASH-friendly kitchen. Plus, they're available year-round.

---

2 small avocados, halved and pitted

2 tablespoons nonfat plain Greek yogurt

Juice of 1 large lemon

¼ teaspoon salt

½ teaspoon freshly ground black pepper

8 large eggs, hard-boiled (see tip), peeled and chopped

3 tablespoons finely chopped fresh dill

3 tablespoons finely chopped fresh parsley

8 whole wheat bread slices (or your choice)

1. Scoop the avocados into a large bowl and mash. Mix in the yogurt, lemon juice, salt, and pepper. Add the eggs, dill, and parsley and combine.
2. Store the bread and salad separately in 4 reusable storage bags and 4 containers and assemble the night before or when serving.
3. To serve, divide the mixture evenly among 4 of the bread slices and top with the other slices to make sandwiches.

- **Storage:** Store in the refrigerator for up to 5 days. Serve chilled or at room temperature.

- **Cooking tip:** For how to hard-boil eggs, see steps 3 to 5 of the step-by-step meal prep in Meal Prep 1 (page 26).

   Per Serving: Calories: 488; Total fat: 22g; Carbohydrates: 48g; Fiber: 8g; Protein: 23g; Calcium: 197mg; Vitamin D: 82 IU; Potassium: 469mg; Magnesium: 32mg; Sodium: 597mg

BREAKFAST HASH

Serves 4
Prep time: 15 minutes • **Cook time:** 25 minutes
GLUTEN-FREE • NUT-FREE • VEGETARIAN OPTION (SEE TIP)

Sweet and salty, this hearty breakfast meal gets a punch of protein from the beef and a high dose of beta-carotene (vitamin A) and fiber from the sweet potatoes and kale. Feel free to change the meat or go meatless—you'll still get delicious results.

Nonstick cooking spray

2 large sweet potatoes, peeled and cut into ½-inch cubes

1 scallion, finely chopped

¼ teaspoon salt

½ teaspoon freshly ground black pepper

8 ounces extra-lean ground beef (96% or leaner)

1 medium onion, diced

2 garlic cloves, minced

1 red bell pepper, diced

¼ teaspoon ground cumin

¼ teaspoon paprika

2 cups coarsely chopped kale leaves

¾ cup shredded reduced-fat Cheddar cheese

4 large eggs

1. Coat a large skillet with cooking spray and heat over medium heat. Add the sweet potatoes, scallion, salt, and pepper. Sauté for 10 minutes, stirring often.
2. Add the beef, onion, garlic, bell pepper, cumin, and paprika. Sauté, stirring frequently, for about 4 minutes, or until the meat browns. Add the kale to the skillet and stir until wilted. Sprinkle with the Cheddar cheese.
3. Make 4 wells in the hash mixture and crack an egg into each. Cover and let the eggs cook until the white is fully cooked and the yolk is to your liking. Divide into 4 storage containers.

- **Storage:** Store in the refrigerator for up to 5 days. To reheat, vent the lid, and microwave on medium for 90 seconds.

- **Variations:** You can use lean ground chicken or turkey instead of beef.

- **Vegetarian option:** Go meatless by swapping in 1 pound of chopped mushrooms for the beef.

Per Serving: Calories: 323; Total fat: 15g; Carbohydrates: 23g; Fiber: 4g; Protein: 25g; Calcium: 273mg; Vitamin D: 44 IU; Potassium: 676mg; Magnesium: 55mg; Sodium: 587mg

HEARTY BREAKFAST CASSEROLE

Serves 4
Prep time: 15 minutes • **Cook time:** 30 minutes
GLUTEN-FREE • NUT-FREE • VEGETARIAN

Hearty and healthy meet in this satisfying casserole: protein-rich eggs, satisfying sweet potato, fresh green veggies, and the umami of mushrooms and cheese all baked together. It can be made ahead, reheats very well, and is a great grab-and-go option for meal prep.

Nonstick cooking spray

1 large green bell pepper, diced

8 ounces cremini mushrooms, diced

½ medium onion, diced

3 garlic cloves, minced

1 large sweet potato, grated

1 cup baby spinach

12 large eggs

3 tablespoons 1% milk

1 teaspoon mustard powder

1 teaspoon paprika

1 teaspoon freshly ground black pepper

½ teaspoon salt

½ cup shredded reduced-fat Colby-Jack cheese

1. Preheat the oven to 350°F. Coat a 9-by-13-inch baking dish with cooking spray.
2. Coat a large skillet with cooking spray and heat over medium heat. Add the bell pepper, mushrooms, onion, garlic, and sweet potato. Sauté, stirring frequently, for 3 to 4 minutes, or until the onion is translucent. Add the spinach and continue to sauté while stirring, until the spinach has wilted. Remove from the heat and set aside to cool slightly.
3. In a large bowl, whisk together the eggs, milk, mustard powder, paprika, black pepper, and salt. Add the sautéed vegetables.
4. Pour the mixture into the prepared baking dish. Bake for 30 minutes. Remove from the oven, sprinkle with the Colby-Jack cheese, return to the oven, and bake for an additional 5 minutes to melt the cheese. Divide into 4 storage containers.

- **Storage:** Store in the refrigerator for up to 5 days. To reheat, vent the lid slightly, and microwave on medium for 2 minutes. The casserole also keeps in the freezer for up to 2 months. To reheat from frozen, microwave on high for 4 minutes.

- **Cooking tip:** This casserole can be frozen uncooked for a fresher taste. Thaw overnight in the refrigerator and then bake as directed in step 4.

- **Variations:** You can add meat to this recipe. Cook 8 ounces of lean ground beef, chicken, or turkey separately, and add it to the egg mixture when you add the sautéed vegetables.

Per Serving: Calories: 378; Total fat: 25g; Carbohydrates: 17g; Fiber: 3g; Protein: 26g; Calcium: 348mg; Vitamin D: 130 IU; Potassium: 717mg; Magnesium: 51mg; Sodium: 658mg

Stuffed Zucchini

Page 114

CHAPTER 4

Sides & Small Plates

LEMON AND HERB COUSCOUS

Serves 6
Prep time: 5 minutes • **Cook time:** 15 minutes
DAIRY-FREE • EGG-FREE • VEGETARIAN OPTION (SEE TIP)

Couscous is a tiny pasta most commonly made of wheat. Whole wheat couscous is always a great choice to increase your whole-grain intake and take steps toward better heart health. This simple citrus-flavored side pairs well with the Savory Pork Loin (page 173) and the Jerk Salmon (page 154).

---

2 cups unsalted chicken stock

1½ cups whole wheat couscous

1 tablespoon finely grated lemon zest

2 tablespoons fresh lemon juice

¼ cup finely chopped fresh parsley

¼ cup finely chopped fresh basil

¼ cup slivered almonds

2 tablespoons extra-virgin olive oil

3 garlic cloves, minced

⅓ cup coarsely chopped fresh chives

1. In a medium saucepan, bring the chicken stock to a boil over high heat. Remove from the heat, stir in the couscous, cover, and let sit for 5 minutes, or until all liquid is absorbed.
2. Stir in the lemon zest, lemon juice, parsley, basil, and almonds. Fluff and mix well with a fork. Set aside.
3. In a large skillet, heat the oil over medium heat. Add the garlic and chives and sauté for about 2 minutes. Add to the couscous mixture and combine well. Divide into 6 storage containers.

- **Storage:** Store in the refrigerator for up to 5 days or in the freezer for up to 1 month. To reheat, vent the lid slightly, and microwave on medium for 2 minutes. To reheat from frozen, microwave on medium for 3 to 4 minutes.

- **Vegetarian option:** Use unsalted vegetable broth.

  Per Serving: Calories: 248; Total fat: 7.5g; Carbohydrates: 36g; Fiber: 6g; Protein: 9g; Calcium: 46mg; Vitamin D: 0 IU; Potassium: 71mg; Magnesium: 16mg; Sodium: 29mg

ROASTED CARROTS AND BEETS

Serves 4
Prep time: 10 minutes • **Cook time:** 1 hour
DAIRY-FREE • EGG-FREE • GLUTEN-FREE • NUT-FREE • VEGAN

Roasting carrots and beets brings out their natural sweetness. It takes a little time, but it's worth the investment. This simple and flavorful dish also packs a nutritional punch: Beets are a superfood, high in folate, vitamin C, potassium, and manganese. Carrots offer more potassium and are an excellent source of beta-carotene (vitamin A). These nutrients lower blood pressure, boost the immune system, and help prevent chronic disease.

Nonstick cooking spray

8 medium carrots, peeled

4 medium beets, peeled

4 tablespoons extra-virgin olive oil, divided

2 tablespoons balsamic vinegar, divided

2 tablespoons chopped fresh parsley, divided

1 teaspoon grated lemon zest

⅛ teaspoon freshly ground black pepper

1. Preheat the oven to 375°F. Line a sheet pan with aluminum foil and coat with nonstick cooking spray.
2. Cut the carrots diagonally into 2-inch lengths on the thin end of the carrot and into 1-inch lengths on the thick end. Cut the beets into 1- to 2-inch cubes.
3. In a large bowl, whisk together 2 tablespoons of oil, 1 tablespoon of vinegar, and 1 tablespoon of parsley. Add the carrots and toss. Place the carrots on half of the prepared sheet pan. Add the remaining 2 tablespoons of oil, 1 tablespoon of vinegar, and 1 tablespoon of parsley to the bowl. Add the beets and toss. Place the beets on the other half of the prepared sheet pan. Sprinkle with the lemon zest and pepper.
4. Bake for about 1 hour, or until the beets turn a dark purple and the carrots a dull orange. They should be soft enough to cut through with a fork. Let cool, then divide into 4 storage containers.

- **Storage:** Store in the refrigerator for up to 5 days. Serve cold or reheat on the stovetop over medium heat with a little bit of water.

- **Variations:** Other vegetables that will caramelize nicely and can be given the same treatment are sweet potatoes, squash, and parsnips.

Per Serving: Calories: 238; Total fat: 18g; Carbohydrates: 21g; Fiber: 6g; Protein: 2g; Calcium: 59mg; Vitamin D: 0 IU; Potassium: 678mg; Magnesium: 35mg; Sodium: 151mg

ZESTY LEMON BRUSSELS SPROUTS

Serves 4

Prep time: 10 minutes • **Cook time:** 35 to 40 minutes

DAIRY-FREE • EGG-FREE • GLUTEN-FREE • NUT-FREE • VEGAN

Brussels sprouts have gone from dreaded side dish to culinary superstar. Much of that has to do with a change to the preparation technique. Boiled is boring. Unseasoned is uninteresting. You must give your sprouts a little time for a great taste. Roasting this dish brings out the caramelized flavors of the Brussels sprouts. Topping with olive oil, black pepper, and lemon zest gives them a little bit of zing.

Nonstick cooking spray

1 pound Brussels sprouts, trimmed and halved

2 tablespoons extra-virgin olive oil

2 tablespoons grated lemon zest

¼ teaspoon freshly ground black pepper

1. Preheat the oven to 400°F. Coat a sheet pan with cooking spray.
2. In a large bowl, toss together the Brussels sprouts, oil, lemon zest, and pepper.
3. Arrange on the prepared sheet pan and roast for 35 to 40 minutes, or until caramelized, shaking the pan every 5 to 7 minutes to ensure they roast evenly. Let cool, then divide into 4 storage containers.

- **Storage:** Store in the refrigerator for up to 5 days or in the freezer for up to 3 months. To reheat, microwave for 30 seconds to 1 minute, roast at 325°F for up to 10 minutes, or sauté in a skillet with a little bit of olive oil until warm. To reheat from frozen, microwave on medium for 2 minutes, or thaw in the refrigerator overnight and follow the refrigerated reheating instructions.

- **Variations:** You can also make this recipe using broccoli or cauliflower, or both. Mix things up by combining all three.

Per Serving: Calories: 162; Total fat: 15g; Carbohydrates: 11g; Fiber: 4.5g; Protein: 4g; Calcium: 52mg; Vitamin D: 0 IU; Potassium: 448mg; Magnesium: 27mg; Sodium: 29mg

CRISP AND SWEET QUINOA

Serves 5
Prep time: 20 minutes · **Cook time:** 20 minutes
DAIRY-FREE · EGG-FREE · GLUTEN-FREE · NUT-FREE · VEGAN

The freshness of cucumber and sweetness of mangos transform this otherwise simple dish. The combination of whole grains, fruit, and a vegetable provide balance. At the same time, quinoa is packed with protein, making this recipe suitable as a main course in its own right. Pair this recipe with Greek Yogurt Dill Dressing (page 184).

---

1 cup quinoa
2 cups water
3 cups diced cucumber
1½ cups diced mango

¼ cup diced onion
½ cup chopped fresh parsley
½ teaspoon freshly ground black pepper

1. If your brand of quinoa has not been prerinsed and washed, place it in a fine-mesh sieve and rinse under cool water for 30 seconds.
2. In a medium saucepan, combine the quinoa and water and bring to a boil. Cover the pot, reduce the heat to a simmer, and cook for 15 to 20 minutes, or until the water has been absorbed and the grain is translucent and tender. If necessary, return to low heat and cook until all the water is absorbed. Let sit for 5 minutes and fluff with a fork.
3. Transfer to a large bowl and let cool for an additional 5 minutes.
4. Add the cucumber, mango, onion, parsley, and pepper. Divide into 5 storage containers.

- **Storage:** Store in the refrigerator for up to 5 days. Serve chilled.

- **Substitution tip:** If mangos are not in season, use canned mangos (drained and rinsed) or thawed frozen mangos.

   Per Serving: Calories: 170; Total fat: 2.5g; Carbohydrates: 32g; Fiber: 4g; Protein: 6g; Calcium: 44mg; Vitamin D: 0 IU; Potassium: 432mg; Magnesium: 86mg; Sodium: 8mg

CILANTRO RICE

Serves 4
Prep time: 5 minutes • **Cook time:** 45 minutes
DAIRY-FREE • EGG-FREE • GLUTEN-FREE • NUT-FREE • VEGAN

Whole grains offer many nutritional benefits, such as fiber for a feeling of fullness, B vitamins for energy, and protein to help you build muscle. Over time, incorporating whole grains can decrease cholesterol, lower blood pressure, regulate blood sugar levels, and improve your digestion. Here, whole-grain rice gets its flavor from a little lime zest and chopped cilantro. Try it with the Beef Tenderloin Medallions with Horseradish Yogurt Sauce (page 178) or the Stuffed Chicken Breasts with Garlic Mushrooms and Zesty Spinach (page 167).

1 tablespoon extra-virgin olive oil
1 cup brown rice
Zest and juice of 1 large lime

1½ cups water
2 tablespoons chopped fresh cilantro

1. In a medium pot, heat the oil over medium heat until warm. Add the rice and lime zest and cook, stirring occasionally, for 3 to 5 minutes, or until toasted.
2. Add the water and bring to a boil. Cover, reduce the heat to low, and simmer for about 45 minutes, or until the rice has absorbed all the water.
3. Stir in the lime juice and cilantro. Divide into 4 storage containers.

- **Storage:** Store in the refrigerator for up to 5 days or in the freezer for up to 3 months. Reheat in the microwave for 1 to 2 minutes. There's no need to thaw before reheating from frozen, but it might need an additional minute in the microwave and stirring halfway through.

- **Substitution tip:** When in a rush, you can use precooked boil-in-a-bag rice, which usually cooks in 10 minutes. Just add the lime zest to the water and cook according to the package directions. Stir in the lime juice and cilantro.

Per Serving: Calories: 202; Total fat: 5g; Carbohydrates: 36g; Fiber: 2g; Protein: 3.5g; Calcium: 6mg; Vitamin D: 0 IU; Potassium: 128mg; Magnesium: 54mg; Sodium: 3mg

JASMINE RICE WITH LEMONGRASS, GARLIC, AND GINGER

Serves 4
Prep time: 5 minutes • **Cook time:** 25 to 30 minutes
DAIRY-FREE • EGG-FREE • GLUTEN-FREE • NUT-FREE • VEGAN

When it comes to rice, it only takes a little to dress it up nice. Here, we focus on a few bright flavors with the lemongrass and ginger, while the garlic provides an earthy contrast. This simple side pairs well with our Zesty Lemon Brussels Sprouts (page 106) and Sesame-Crusted Ahi Tuna Steaks (page 152). Put all three together and you have one delicious and balanced dinner.

2 teaspoons extra-virgin olive oil
½ lemongrass stalk, halved lengthwise
   and pounded
1-inch piece fresh ginger, peeled

1 garlic clove, minced
1 cup jasmine rice
1 cup water
1 scallion, thinly sliced (optional)

1. In a small saucepan, heat the oil over medium heat. Add the lemongrass and ginger and cook for 1 minute. Toss in the garlic and cook for another minute.
2. Pour in the rice and water and bring to a boil. Reduce the heat to a simmer, cover, and cook for 25 to 30 minutes, or until all the water is absorbed and the rice is tender. Let rest for 5 minutes.
3. Fluff with a fork. Discard the lemongrass and ginger. Let cool, then divide into 4 storage containers. Top each with sliced scallion (if using).

- **Storage:** Store in the refrigerator for up to 5 days or in the freezer for up to 3 months. To reheat, microwave for 1 to 2 minutes with a glass of water next to it to maintain moisture. To reheat from frozen, microwave on medium for 3 to 4 minutes.

- **Variations:** Brown rice is an easy swap here. You will need to cook the rice a little bit longer, but you'll gain fiber, energy-producing B vitamins, and protein.

Per Serving: Calories: 181; Total fat: 2g; Carbohydrates: 36g; Fiber: 0g; Protein: 3g; Calcium: 1mg; Vitamin D: 0 IU; Potassium: 3mg; Magnesium: 0mg; Sodium: 0mg

THREE-BEAN SALAD

Serves 6
Prep time: 5 minutes • **Cook time:** 5 minutes
DAIRY-FREE • EGG-FREE • GLUTEN-FREE • NUT-FREE • VEGAN

A summer favorite—take this salad to a potluck, barbecue, or picnic, and add color and great taste to any food table. Making this fiber- and iron-rich salad could not be easier. It pairs well with the Pineapple and Shrimp Skewers (page 149) or next to the Breaded and Baked Chicken Tenders (page 166).

1 (15-ounce) can no-salt-added green beans, drained

1 (15-ounce) can no-salt-added chickpeas, drained and rinsed

1 (15-ounce) can no-salt-added kidney beans, drained and rinsed

1 medium red onion, cut into thin rings

2 celery stalks, finely chopped

¾ cup finely chopped fresh parsley

¼ cup sugar

½ cup apple cider vinegar

3 tablespoons extra-virgin olive oil

½ teaspoon salt

½ teaspoon freshly ground black pepper

1. In a large bowl, toss together the green beans, chickpeas, kidney beans, onion, celery, and parsley.
2. In a small bowl, whisk together the sugar, vinegar, oil, salt, and pepper. Add this to the bean mixture and toss to coat thoroughly. Divide into 6 storage containers.

- **Storage:** Store in the refrigerator for up to 7 days. Let it come nearly to room temperature before serving.

- **Substitution tip:** If you are having trouble finding no-salt-added canned beans, you can use low-sodium or reduced-sodium canned beans, but make sure to drain and rinse them before using.

Per Serving: Calories: 251; Total fat: 7.5g; Carbohydrates: 37g; Fiber: 10g; Protein: 10g; Calcium: 103mg; Vitamin D: 0 IU; Potassium: 421mg; Magnesium: 54mg; Sodium: 318mg

MASHED SWEET POTATOES

Serves 4

Prep time: 15 minutes • **Cook time:** 25 minutes

EGG-FREE • GLUTEN-FREE • NUT-FREE • VEGETARIAN

Creamy and rich, these mashed sweet potatoes will melt in your mouth. A rich source of beta-carotene (vitamin A), vitamin C, and fiber, this recipe provides a healthier alternative to your standard meat-and-potato side dish. Try it with the Pistachio-Crusted Tilapia (page 156) and the Barbecue Turkey Breast (page 170).

---

6 medium sweet potatoes, peeled and cubed

2 tablespoons unsalted butter

¼ cup nonfat plain Greek yogurt

1 teaspoon freshly ground black pepper

¼ teaspoon salt

⅓ cup 1% milk

¼ cup thinly sliced scallions

¼ cup finely chopped fresh parsley

1 garlic clove, minced

1. In a large saucepan, combine the sweet potatoes and enough water to cover them by 1 inch. Bring to a boil, then reduce the heat to a simmer and cook for 10 to 15 minutes, or until the sweet potatoes are tender.
2. Drain well and return the sweet potatoes to the saucepan. Add the butter, yogurt, pepper, and salt. With a hand mixer, a potato masher, or a fork, blend while slowly adding the milk, until the ingredients are mixed. Add the scallions, parsley, and garlic and mix until well combined. Let cool, then divide into 4 storage containers.

- **Storage:** Store in the refrigerator for up to 5 days or in the freezer for up to 3 months. To reheat, vent the lid slightly, and microwave on medium for 2 minutes. If frozen, microwave on medium for 5 minutes, stirring halfway through.

- **Ingredient tip:** To save time and effort, you can purchase frozen sweet potato cubes.

Per Serving: Calories: 242; Total fat: 6g; Carbohydrates: 42g; Fiber: 6.5g; Protein: 6g; Calcium: 116mg; Vitamin D: 10 IU; Potassium: 760mg; Magnesium: 57mg; Sodium: 271mg

SUMMER RAINBOW PASTA SALAD

Serves 8

Prep time: 10 minutes • **Cook time:** 15 minutes

EGG-FREE • NUT-FREE • VEGETARIAN • GLUTEN-FREE OPTION (SEE TIP)

This pasta—with its delicate citrus sauce, crowd-pleasing peas, and fresh mint—can be served hot or cold. It's topped with a little bit of Parmesan cheese to add a nutty tang. This dish is also quick and easy, making it a great side for a weeknight meal. With just a few ingredients, it's budget friendly as well.

1½ cups frozen peas

8 ounces rainbow rotini pasta

¼ cup extra-virgin olive oil

Zest and juice of 2 lemons

1 garlic clove, minced

½ cup grated Parmesan cheese

¼ cup chopped fresh mint

1. Bring a large pot of water to a boil. Add the peas and cook for about 3 minutes, or until tender. With a slotted spoon, transfer the peas to a large bowl and set aside.
2. Add the pasta to the boiling water and cook until al dente according to the package directions. Drain the pasta and let cool to room temperature.
3. Meanwhile, to the bowl of peas, add the oil, lemon zest, lemon juice, garlic, Parmesan cheese, and mint.
4. Add the pasta to the bowl and combine well. Divide into 8 storage containers.

- **Storage:** Store in the refrigerator for up to 5 days or in the freezer for up to 1 month. Reheat for 1 to 2 minutes in the microwave, or serve cold. If frozen, thaw in the refrigerator overnight.

- **Gluten-free option:** Use gluten-free pasta.

  Per Serving: Calories: 205; Total fat: 9g; Carbohydrates: 26g; Fiber: 2g; Protein: 7g; Calcium: 54mg; Vitamin D: 1 IU; Potassium: 57mg; Magnesium: 9mg; Sodium: 116mg

SWEET POTATOES WITH CHOPPED PISTACHIOS

Serves 4
Prep time: 10 minutes • **Cook time:** 45 minutes
EGG-FREE • GLUTEN-FREE • VEGETARIAN • NUT-FREE OPTION (SEE TIP)

Pistachios are an excellent source of protein, fiber, thiamin, and vitamin B_6. They also provide calcium, riboflavin, folate, vitamin B_5, and vitamins E and K. All these nutrients work together to keep your circulatory, skeletal, and digestive systems healthy while lowering blood pressure. These nutritious nuts are a perfect addition to sweet potatoes, which are rich in potassium, beta-carotene (vitamin A), and fiber.

Nonstick cooking spray (optional)
4 large sweet potatoes, peeled and cut into
　1-inch cubes
4 tablespoons extra-virgin olive oil, divided
¼ teaspoon freshly ground black pepper
¼ cup finely chopped pistachios

½ teaspoon ground cumin
½ teaspoon ground turmeric
Pinch ground cinnamon
Pinch red pepper flakes (optional)
1 cup nonfat plain Greek yogurt

1. Preheat the oven to 375°F. Line a sheet pan with aluminum foil or coat with nonstick cooking spray.
2. In a large bowl, toss the sweet potatoes with 2 tablespoons of oil and the pepper. Spread onto the prepared sheet pan and roast for 30 to 35 minutes, or until crispy. Remove from the oven.
3. In a large skillet, heat the remaining 2 tablespoons of oil until warm. Add the pistachios, cumin, turmeric, cinnamon, and pepper flakes (if using) and stir until well combined. Add the roasted sweet potatoes, stir to coat, and remove from the heat.
4. Divide the sweet potato and pistachio mixture into 4 storage containers. Store the yogurt separately. When ready to serve, spread the yogurt out onto a serving platter. Top with the sweet potato and pistachio mixture.

- **Storage:** Store in the refrigerator for up to 5 days or in the freezer for up to 3 months. Reheat for 1 to 2 minutes in the microwave if refrigerated; 4 minutes if frozen.

- **Nut-free option:** Use sunflower seeds instead of pistachios.

   Per Serving: Calories: 328; Total fat: 17g; Carbohydrates: 34g; Fiber: 5.5g; Protein: 10g; Calcium: 122mg; Vitamin D: 0 IU; Potassium: 669mg; Magnesium: 52mg; Sodium: 137mg

STUFFED ZUCCHINI

Serves 6
Prep time: 10 minutes • **Cook time:** 35 minutes
EGG-FREE • GLUTEN-FREE • NUT-FREE • VEGETARIAN OPTION (SEE TIP)

Stuffed squash or zucchini originally comes from Mediterranean and Middle Eastern cuisines. When stuffed with meat, as in this dish, these vegetables are served hot as a main course. When meatless, they tend to be served warm or at room temperature as a side dish. Whichever way you choose, you can't go wrong with this recipe.

3 large zucchini

Nonstick cooking spray

8 ounces ground chicken

1 medium onion, diced

2 garlic cloves, minced

6 ounces mushrooms, coarsely chopped

2 cups Simple Tomato Sauce (page 187) or
 store-bought no-salt-added pasta sauce

1 large tomato, diced

1 medium red bell pepper, diced

1 teaspoon dried oregano

¼ teaspoon salt

½ teaspoon freshly ground black pepper

¾ cup shredded part-skim low-moisture
 mozzarella cheese

1. Preheat the oven to 375°F.
2. Halve the zucchini lengthwise and scoop out the seeds and some of the flesh to turn them into "boats" and make room for the stuffing. Place the zucchini, cut-side up, in a large baking dish.
3. Coat a large skillet with cooking spray and heat over medium-high heat. Add the chicken, onion, and garlic and cook and stir for 2 to 3 minutes. Add the mushrooms and continue to stir until the mushrooms have stopped releasing liquid and the chicken has browned.
4. Stir in the tomato sauce, diced tomato, bell pepper, oregano, salt, and black pepper. Reduce the heat to a simmer and cook for 5 to 8 minutes to thicken slightly and blend the flavors. Remove from the heat.
5. Distribute the mixture evenly among the zucchini boats. Top each zucchini boat with 2 tablespoons of mozzarella cheese.
6. Bake for 20 to 25 minutes, or until the zucchini has softened and the cheese is starting to brown. Let cool, then divide the zucchini boats among 6 storage containers.

- **Storage:** Store in the refrigerator for up to 5 days. To reheat, vent the lid slightly, and micro-wave on medium for 2 minutes.

- **Vegetarian option:** Skip the chicken, and double up on the mushrooms.

Per Serving: Calories: 266; Total fat: 17g; Carbohydrates: 21g; Fiber: 4g; Protein: 15g; Calcium: 147mg; Vitamin D: 1 IU; Potassium: 703mg; Magnesium: 41mg; Sodium: 347mg

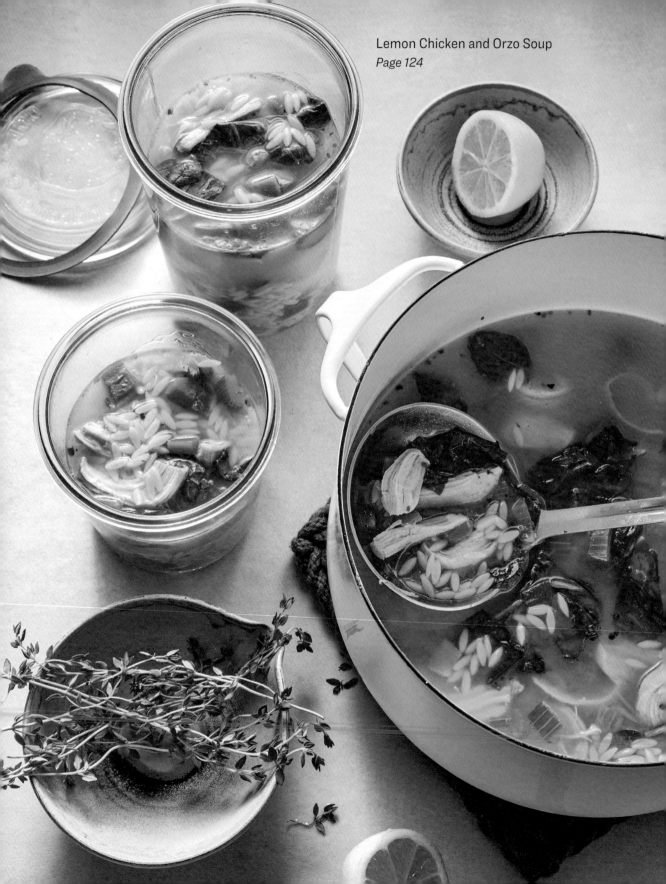

Lemon Chicken and Orzo Soup
Page 124

CHAPTER 5

Salads & Soups

SIMPLE GREEN SALAD

Serves 4
Prep time: 5 minutes • **Cook time:** 5 minutes
EGG-FREE • GLUTEN-FREE • NUT-FREE • VEGETARIAN • DAIRY-FREE/VEGAN OPTION (SEE TIP)

Simple ingredients and a delicious combination of tart flavors make this salad a great addition to any meal. The nice crunch of the cucumber and onion tells you this is not your typical green salad, and the Parmesan cheese works well with the acidity of the lemon juice. This dish pairs nicely with the Mushroom Bolognese (page 139), the Sesame-Crusted Ahi Tuna Steaks (page 152), and the Honey-Garlic Pork Chops (page 174).

¼ cup extra-virgin olive oil

2 tablespoons fresh lemon juice

¼ teaspoon salt

¼ teaspoon freshly ground black pepper

6 cups loosely packed mixed greens

½ small red onion, thinly sliced

1 small cucumber, peeled and thinly sliced

¼ cup shredded Parmesan cheese

1. In a small bowl, whisk together the oil, lemon juice, salt, and pepper until well combined. Store the dressing in 4 condiment cups.
2. In a large bowl, combine the mixed greens, onion, and cucumber. Divide the salad into 4 medium storage containers. Top each with 1 tablespoon of Parmesan cheese.
3. To serve, toss the dressing and salad together.

- **Storage:** Store in the refrigerator for up to 5 days.

- **Dairy-free/vegan option:** Skip the Parmesan cheese but add ¼ cup of sunflower seeds for texture.

  Per Serving: Calories: 162; Total fat: 15g; Carbohydrates: 6g; Fiber: 2g; Protein: 3g; Calcium: 96mg; Vitamin D: 1 IU; Potassium: 84mg; Magnesium: 8mg; Sodium: 290mg

KALE-POPPY SEED SALAD

Serves 6
Prep time: 10 minutes • **Cook time:** 5 minutes
EGG-FREE • GLUTEN-FREE • NUT-FREE • VEGETARIAN

This is Maria-Paula's favorite salad. The crunch of the pumpkin seeds combined with the sweetness of the cranberries is the perfect addition to crispy, fresh kale. Kale is an excellent source of beta-carotene (vitamin A) and vitamins C and K. And it is a good source of calcium, magnesium, and potassium, making it a perfect DASH food.

½ cup nonfat plain Greek yogurt
2 tablespoons apple cider vinegar
½ tablespoon extra-virgin olive oil
1 teaspoon poppy seeds
1 teaspoon sugar

4 cups firmly packed finely chopped kale
2 cups broccoli slaw
2 cups thinly sliced Brussels sprouts
6 tablespoons dried cranberries
6 tablespoons hulled pumpkin seeds

1. In a small bowl, whisk together the yogurt, vinegar, oil, poppy seeds, and sugar until well combined. Store the dressing in 6 condiment cups.
2. In a large bowl, mix together the kale, broccoli slaw, and Brussels sprouts. Divide the greens into 6 large storage containers and top each salad with cranberries and pumpkin seeds.
3. To serve, toss the greens with the poppy seed dressing to coat.

- **Storage:** Store in the refrigerator for up to 5 days.

- **Substitution tip:** You can use store-bought poppy seed dressing, but mix it with equal parts plain nonfat Greek yogurt. Make sure you limit it to 2 tablespoons per serving.

Per Serving: Calories: 129; Total fat: 6g; Carbohydrates: 13g; Fiber: 3g; Protein: 8g; Calcium: 72mg; Vitamin D: 0 IU; Potassium: 257mg; Magnesium: 68mg; Sodium: 26mg

WEDGE SALAD WITH CREAMY BLUE CHEESE DRESSING

Serves 4
Prep time: 15 minutes
EGG-FREE • GLUTEN-FREE • VEGETARIAN

Adding more nutrition to a classic wedge salad is easy. Here, iceberg lettuce—the typical wedge salad lettuce—is replaced with romaine, which provides the carotenoids beta-carotene (vitamin A), lutein, and zeaxanthin—all nutrients that protect your eyes. Romaine lettuce also contains vitamin K, an essential nutrient in blood clotting and regulating insulin. The almonds, Greek yogurt, and blue cheese add protein. The blue cheese also adds just the right tang without excess salt.

1 cup nonfat plain Greek yogurt

Juice of ½ large lemon

¼ teaspoon freshly ground black pepper

¼ teaspoon salt

⅓ cup crumbled blue cheese

2 heads romaine lettuce, stem end trimmed, halved lengthwise

1 cup grape tomatoes, halved

½ cup slivered almonds

1. In a small bowl, whisk together the yogurt, lemon juice, pepper, salt, and blue cheese until well combined. Store the dressing in 4 condiment cups.
2. Divide the lettuce halves and tomatoes among 4 large storage containers. Store the almonds separately.
3. To serve, arrange a half-head of romaine on a plate and top with the grape tomatoes. Sprinkle with 2 tablespoons of almonds and drizzle with the salad dressing.

- **Storage:** Store in the refrigerator for up to 5 days.

  Per Serving: Calories: 216; Total fat: 11g; Carbohydrates: 20g; Fiber: 9g; Protein: 16g; Calcium: 267mg; Vitamin D: 2 IU; Potassium: 995mg; Magnesium: 90mg; Sodium: 329mg

SOUTHWESTERN BEAN SALAD WITH CREAMY AVOCADO DRESSING

Serves 4

Prep time: 15 minutes

EGG-FREE • GLUTEN-FREE • NUT-FREE • VEGETARIAN

This Southwestern salad is the perfect blend of delicious and nutritious. The meaty and satisfying black beans contain protective folate, antioxidants, and essential minerals, including manganese, magnesium, and iron. The crunchy lettuce, corn, and juicy tomatoes bring not only great flavor and texture, but also plenty of potassium and fiber. And the creamy cilantro-flecked avocado and yogurt dressing offers healthy fats and high-quality protein.

1 head romaine lettuce, chopped

1 (15-ounce) can no-salt-added black beans, drained and rinsed

2 cups fresh or (thawed) frozen corn kernels

2 cups grape tomatoes, halved

2 small avocados, halved and pitted

1 cup chopped fresh cilantro

1 cup nonfat plain Greek yogurt

8 scallions, chopped

3 garlic cloves, quartered

Zest and juice of 1 large lime

½ teaspoon sugar

1. In a large bowl, combine the lettuce, beans, corn, and tomatoes. Toss until well combined. Divide the salad into 4 large storage containers.
2. Scoop the avocado flesh into a blender or food processor. Add the cilantro, yogurt, scallions, garlic, lime zest and juice, and sugar. Blend until well combined. Divide the dressing into 4 condiment cups.
3. To serve, toss the salad and the dressing together.

- **Storage:** Store in the refrigerator for up to 5 days.

- **Substitution tip:** Use no-salt-added canned corn if fresh or frozen are not available.

Per Serving: Calories: 349; Total fat: 11g; Carbohydrates: 53g; Fiber: 16g; Protein: 19g; Calcium: 210mg; Vitamin D: 0 IU; Potassium: 1,277mg; Magnesium: 118mg; Sodium: 77mg

COBB PASTA SALAD

Serves 6
Prep time: 20 minutes • **Cook time:** 10 minutes
NUT-FREE • GLUTEN-FREE OPTION (SEE TIP)

Colorful, flavorful, and simple, this salad might be your new go-to lunch favorite. It's a nicely balanced meal with something from every food group—not to mention it's high in fiber and protein and rich in potassium and magnesium.

1 pound whole wheat rotini pasta

2 cups chopped cooked chicken breast (about 3 breasts)

8 low-sodium turkey bacon slices, cooked and chopped

4 scallions, sliced

1½ cups cherry tomatoes, halved

¼ teaspoon freshly ground black pepper

4 hard-boiled eggs, peeled and coarsely chopped

⅓ cup crumbled blue cheese

1 cup frozen avocado cubes

¾ cup Greek Yogurt Dill Dressing (page 184)

1. In a large pot of boiling water, cook the pasta until al dente according to the package directions. Rinse under cold water, then drain.
2. In a large bowl, combine the pasta, chicken, bacon, scallions, tomatoes, and pepper. Toss until well combined.
3. Add the eggs and blue cheese and fold until mixed well. Divide the salad into 6 storage containers. Divide the avocado into 6 small storage containers.
4. Make the dressing as directed and store in 6 condiment cups.
5. The night before you're planning on having a salad, add the portion of frozen avocado to the salad so they will be soft by mealtime the next day. Serve drizzled with the dressing.

- **Storage:** Store the salad and dressing in the refrigerator for up to 5 days. Store the avocado in the freezer.

- **Ingredient tip:** If you don't have access to frozen avocado, don't slice into your avocado until the day you plan to serve the salad.

- **Gluten-free option:** Use gluten-free pasta.

  Per Serving: Calories: 550; Total fat: 18g; Carbohydrates: 62g; Fiber: 9.5g; Protein: 40g; Calcium: 128mg; Vitamin D: 31 IU; Potassium: 918mg; Magnesium: 139mg; Sodium: 619mg

TOMATO-BASIL SOUP

Serves 4

Prep time: 5 minutes • **Cook time:** 30 minutes

EGG-FREE • GLUTEN-FREE • NUT-FREE • VEGETARIAN • DAIRY-FREE/VEGAN OPTION (SEE TIP)

This healthy classic soup is easy to make from scratch. Tomatoes are a major source of lycopene, an antioxidant that has been linked to reduced risk of heart disease and cancer. This soup is also a great source of potassium. This is a DASH favorite—its flavorful simplicity is sure to please both kids and adults.

---

3 tablespoons extra-virgin olive oil

1 large onion, diced

3 garlic cloves, minced

2½ pounds roma (plum) tomatoes, cut into big chunks

½ teaspoon salt

1 teaspoon freshly ground black pepper

10 large fresh basil leaves

⅓ cup 1% milk

1. In a medium saucepan, heat the oil over medium heat. Add the onion and garlic and sauté for 8 minutes, stirring often. Add the tomatoes, increase the heat, and cook, stirring frequently, for about 15 minutes, or until the tomatoes soften, change in color, and start breaking apart. Remove from the heat. Stir in the salt, pepper, and basil and let sit for 3 to 5 minutes.

2. Working in batches if necessary, pour the mixture into a blender. Open the steam vent in the blender lid and puree on low, slowly pouring the milk in, a little bit at a time, until a smooth consistency is achieved. Let cool before dividing among 4 storage containers.

- **Storage:** Store in the refrigerator for up to 5 days or in the freezer for up to 3 months. To reheat, vent the lid slightly, and microwave on medium for 2 minutes. To reheat from the freezer, thaw in the refrigerator overnight, then follow the refrigerated instructions.

- **Dairy-free/vegan option:** Use soy milk instead of cow's milk.

Per Serving: Calories: 165; Total fat: 11g; Carbohydrates: 16g; Fiber: 4g; Protein: 3g; Calcium: 69mg; Vitamin D: 10 IU; Potassium: 717mg; Magnesium: 37mg; Sodium: 315mg

LEMON CHICKEN AND ORZO SOUP

Serves 4

Prep time: 10 minutes • **Cook time:** 40 minutes

DAIRY-FREE • EGG-FREE • NUT-FREE • GLUTEN-FREE OPTION (SEE TIP)

One of the places sodium tends to hide is in cans of soups. Taking a little time to make soup at home can help you moderate your sodium intake. Here, a traditional chicken soup is remade with a few Mediterranean flavors such as thyme, oregano, and lemon. It's a crowd-pleaser all around.

2 ounces orzo pasta

12 ounces boneless, skinless chicken breast

6 cups unsalted chicken stock, divided

1 tablespoon extra-virgin olive oil

2 medium carrots, diced

2 celery stalks, diced

½ medium onion, diced

1 garlic clove, minced

½ teaspoon dried thyme

½ teaspoon dried oregano

¼ teaspoon freshly ground black pepper

1 bay leaf

Zest and juice of 1 large lemon

2 cups spinach leaves

1. Bring a large pot of water to a boil. Add the pasta and cook until al dente according to the package directions. Drain.
2. Meanwhile, in a small pot, combine the chicken and 2 cups of chicken stock. Bring to a boil, then quickly reduce the heat to a simmer, partially cover, and cook for 5 to 10 minutes, or until the chicken is no longer pink in the center. Remove from the heat and let stand in the hot chicken stock for 20 minutes.
3. In a stockpot, heat the oil over medium-high heat. Add the carrots, celery, and onion and cook for 5 to 7 minutes, or until the vegetables have softened and the onion is translucent. Add the garlic and cook for 1 minute. Season with the thyme, oregano, and pepper. Add the bay leaf and remaining 4 cups of chicken stock and bring the mixture to a boil. Partially cover, reduce the heat, and simmer for 10 minutes.
4. Add the lemon zest, lemon juice, drained orzo, and spinach to the soup. Shred the chicken and add it to the soup. Continue to cook for 2 to 3 minutes, or until the spinach is wilted. Remove the bay leaf. Divide the soup among 4 storage containers.

- **Storage:** Store in the refrigerator for up to 5 days or in the freezer for up to 3 months. Reheat for 1 to 2 minutes in the microwave, stirring once. If reheating from frozen, microwave on medium for 4 minutes.

- **Gluten-free option:** Use gluten-free orzo.

  Per Serving: Calories: 275; Total fat: 6.5g; Carbohydrates: 23g; Fiber: 4.5g; Protein: 32g; Calcium: 191mg; Vitamin D: 1 IU; Potassium: 622mg; Magnesium: 64mg; Sodium: 196mg

BUTTERNUT SQUASH SOUP

Serves 4
Prep time: 10 minutes • **Cook time:** 55 minutes
EGG-FREE • GLUTEN-FREE • NUT-FREE • VEGETARIAN

Prepping butternut squash can be lots of work. Roasting it first helps with the problem of peeling it. Less than an hour in the oven caramelizes the squash while allowing for easy scooping from the peel. The roast time also benefits the garlic, bringing out an intense smoky flavor for your soup.

Nonstick cooking spray (optional)
½ medium red onion, cut into wedges
3 garlic cloves, peeled
6 teaspoons extra-virgin olive oil, divided
⅜ teaspoon freshly ground black
  pepper, divided

1 large (3-pound) butternut squash, halved
  and seeded
½ teaspoon ground cinnamon
⅛ teaspoon ground nutmeg
3 cups unsalted vegetable broth
½ cup nonfat plain Greek yogurt

1. Preheat the oven to 400°F. Line a sheet pan with aluminum foil or coat with nonstick cooking spray.
2. In a small bowl, toss the onion and garlic with 2 teaspoons of oil and ⅛ teaspoon of pepper. Spread them onto the prepared sheet pan. Brush the cut sides of the butternut squash with the remaining 4 teaspoons of oil and sprinkle with the remaining ¼ teaspoon of pepper. Place the squash, cut-side up, on the prepared sheet pan.
3. Roast for 20 minutes, turning the garlic once, and remove the garlic cloves. Allow the onion wedges and squash to cook for an additional 30 to 35 minutes, or until the squash is fork-tender.
4. Let the squash cool slightly, for about 10 minutes, then spoon the squash out of the skin into a blender. Or if you have an immersion blender, spoon the squash into a large pot.
5. To the blender or pot, add the onion, garlic, cinnamon, nutmeg, and vegetable broth. Blend until smooth. (If made in a blender, pour the soup into a pot.)
6. Heat the pot of soup over medium heat until warm.
7. Remove from the heat and stir in the yogurt, 1 tablespoon at a time to avoid curdling. Divide the soup into 4 storage containers.

- **Storage:** Store in the refrigerator for up to 5 days or in the freezer for up to 3 months. Reheat from the refrigerator for 1 to 2 minutes in the microwave, stirring once. If frozen, reheat in the microwave for 5 to 6 minutes, stirring once.

- **Ingredient tip:** You can find butternut squash in cubes in the produce section in some grocery stores. Purchase about 2½ pounds. If fresh, toss with onion, garlic, oil, and pepper. Spread out onto the sheet pan and roast for 40 minutes. The onion still may need to cook a little longer until tender. The freezer section is usually a safe bet if it's not available fresh. Cook time is the same whether fresh or frozen. Preheat the sheet pan to help speed up the process.

Per Serving: Calories: 231; Total fat: 7g; Carbohydrates: 40g; Fiber: 7g; Protein: 7g; Calcium: 182mg; Vitamin D: 0 IU; Potassium: 1,080mg; Magnesium: 103mg; Sodium: 41mg

CREAM OF CAULIFLOWER SOUP

Serves 5
Prep time: 10 minutes • **Cook time:** 25 minutes
EGG-FREE • NUT-FREE • VEGETARIAN OPTION (SEE TIP)

A quick preparation and budget-friendly ingredients make this soup hit the spot. Its mild flavor and creamy comfort satisfy even the pickiest palates. Cauliflower is rich in fiber and contains carotenoid and flavonoid antioxidants, which may reduce the risk of heart disease.

---

2 tablespoons extra-virgin olive oil

1 large head cauliflower, stemmed and chopped

3 garlic cloves, minced

2 tablespoons dried thyme

1 medium onion, diced

2½ cups unsalted chicken stock

½ teaspoon salt

1 teaspoon freshly ground black pepper

2 tablespoons unsalted butter

2 tablespoons whole wheat flour

2½ cups 1% milk

¼ cup grated Parmesan cheese

1. In a large pot, heat the oil over medium-high heat. Add the cauliflower, garlic, thyme, and onion and sauté for about 2 minutes, stirring regularly. Stir in the chicken stock, salt, and pepper. Bring to a boil, then reduce the heat to a simmer and cook for about 20 minutes, or until the vegetables soften.

2. Meanwhile, in a medium saucepan, melt the butter over medium heat. Add the flour and whisk for 2 minutes until well mixed. Continue to whisk and start adding the milk. Bring to a light boil while continuing to stir, then remove from the heat. Add the Parmesan cheese and whisk again.

3. Pour the Parmesan cream sauce into the cauliflower and broth mixture and stir until well combined. Let cool, then divide the soup into 5 storage containers.

- **Storage:** Store in the refrigerator for up to 5 days or in the freezer for up to 3 months. To reheat, vent the lid slightly, and microwave on medium for 2 minutes. To reheat from the freezer, vent the lid slightly, and microwave on medium for 5 minutes.

- **Cooking tip:** For a creamier texture, blend the cauliflower to your desired consistency. Then fold in the Parmesan cream sauce.

- **Vegetarian option:** Use vegetable broth.

  Per Serving: Calories: 240; Total fat: 13g; Carbohydrates: 21g; Fiber: 4.5g; Protein: 12g; Calcium: 269mg; Vitamin D: 59 IU; Potassium: 760mg; Magnesium: 50mg; Sodium: 446mg

CHICKEN-POTATO SOUP

Serves 4
Prep time: 15 minutes • **Cook time:** 25 minutes
EGG-FREE • NUT-FREE • GLUTEN-FREE OPTION (SEE TIP)

This hearty and comforting soup is the perfect choice for a cold night. It's also rich in protein and calcium thanks to the chicken, milk, and Cheddar cheese. What we love most is its simplicity.

2½ tablespoons unsalted butter

½ medium onion, diced

2 small carrots, diced

2 celery stalks, diced

1 teaspoon dried thyme

2½ tablespoons whole wheat flour

2 cups unsalted chicken stock

1½ cups 1% milk, plus more as needed

2 medium Russet potatoes, peeled and cubed

1½ cups diced cooked chicken breast

1 cup shredded reduced-fat sharp
  Cheddar cheese

¼ teaspoon salt

½ teaspoon freshly ground black pepper

2 tablespoons chopped fresh parsley

1. In a large saucepan, melt the butter over medium heat. Add the onion, carrots, and celery and sauté for about 3 minutes, or until tender. Add the thyme and sauté for an additional minute, or until fragrant.
2. Add the flour and whisk for about 1 minute, or until it is lightly browned. Little by little, start adding the chicken stock and milk, whisking constantly until it is mixed in and starts thickening.
3. Add the potatoes. Bring to a boil, then reduce the heat to a simmer and cook for 10 to 15 minutes, or until the potatoes are tender. Add the chicken and slowly add the Cheddar cheese, whisking for 1 to 2 minutes, or until the mixture is smooth. Add the salt, pepper, and parsley. If the consistency is too thick for your liking, add additional milk. Divide the soup into 4 storage containers.

- **Storage:** Store in the refrigerator for up to 5 days or in the freezer for up to 3 months. To reheat, vent the lid slightly, and microwave on medium for 2 minutes. To reheat from frozen, vent the lid slightly, and microwave on medium for 5 minutes, stirring halfway through.

- **Gluten-free option:** Use gluten-free all-purpose flour.

  Per Serving: Calories: 394; Total fat: 16g; Carbohydrates: 27g; Fiber: 3g; Protein: 36g; Calcium: 431mg; Vitamin D: 51 IU; Potassium: 824mg; Magnesium: 66mg; Sodium: 509mg

Tomato and Basil Pizzas
Page 132

Vegetarian Mains

TOMATO AND BASIL PIZZAS

Makes 2 pizzas (3 servings each)
Prep time: 5 minutes • **Cook time:** 12 to 15 minutes
EGG-FREE • NUT-FREE

Everyone loves pizza, but restaurant pies tend to be loaded with salt. Here, we've reduced the sodium with a homemade sauce and a less salty crust. Market Pantry, Simply Balanced Organic, and Flatzza are great reduced-sodium crust options. (Look for one that has less than 140 milligrams of sodium.) Want to enhance the healthiness even further? Load it up with vegetables, such as mushrooms, bell pepper, onions, or spinach.

Nonstick cooking spray (optional)
2 tablespoons extra-virgin olive oil
2 garlic cloves, minced
½ medium red onion, finely chopped
2 teaspoons dried oregano
2 teaspoons dried basil
½ teaspoon freshly ground black pepper

2 cups no-salt-added tomato sauce
¼ cup no-salt-added tomato paste
2 (12- or 14-inch) reduced-sodium prebaked pizza crusts
2 cups shredded part-skim low-moisture mozzarella cheese, divided
2 cups fresh basil leaves, chopped

1. Preheat the oven to 400°F. Line a sheet pan with foil or coat with cooking spray.
2. In a medium skillet, heat the oil over low heat. Add the garlic and onion and stir for 1 minute, or until fragrant. Add the oregano, basil, pepper, tomato sauce, and tomato paste. Simmer for 10 minutes.
3. Place 1 of the pizza crusts on the prepared sheet pan. Top with half of the sauce. Sprinkle on 1 cup of mozzarella cheese.
4. Bake for 12 to 15 minutes, or until the crust is lightly browned and the cheese is melted. Allow to cool for 3 to 5 minutes before cutting into 3 wedges. Repeat with the other pizza crust, remaining sauce, and 1 cup of mozzarella cheese to make the second pizza.
5. Divide among 6 reusable bags. Store the basil in a separate container. When reheating, top each wedge with ⅓ cup of basil.

• **Storage:** Store in the refrigerator for up to 5 days. To reheat, microwave for 1 to 2 minutes, or bake at 325°F for up to 10 minutes.

Per Serving: Calories: 278; Total fat: 15g; Carbohydrates: 27g; Fiber: 6g; Protein: 15g; Calcium: 245mg; Vitamin D: 6 IU; Potassium: 269mg; Magnesium: 19mg; Sodium: 444mg

COUSCOUS AND CHICKPEA BOWLS WITH TAHINI SAUCE

Serves 3

Prep time: 10 minutes • **Cook time:** 15 minutes

DAIRY-FREE • EGG-FREE • NUT-FREE • GLUTEN-FREE OPTION (SEE TIP) • VEGAN OPTION (SEE TIP)

The main ingredients in this dish—couscous, chickpeas, and tahini—give it a strong Middle Eastern flair. They're also rich in fiber and provide a balanced source of proteins, making this recipe a superb choice when looking for a weekday meatless meal.

⅓ cup tahini

Juice of 2 large lemons

1 teaspoon honey

3 tablespoons extra-virgin olive oil, divided

2 tablespoons water, plus 1¼ cups

2 (15-ounce) cans no-salt-added chickpeas, drained and rinsed

½ teaspoon ground cumin

½ teaspoon freshly ground black pepper

1 cup whole wheat couscous

¼ cup finely chopped fresh parsley

2 small cucumbers, peeled and chopped

1 pint cherry tomatoes, halved

1 large green bell pepper, chopped

1 medium onion, chopped

1. In a small bowl, whisk together the tahini, lemon juice, honey, and 1 tablespoon of oil. Whisk in 2 tablespoons of water until the mixture is creamy. Set aside.
2. In a medium bowl, stir together the chickpeas, 1 tablespoon of oil, the cumin, and black pepper.
3. In a medium saucepan, bring the remaining 1¼ cups of water to a boil. Add the couscous and return to a boil. Remove from the heat and let rest for 5 minutes. Fluff with the remaining 1 tablespoon of oil and the parsley.
4. In a large bowl, combine the cucumbers, tomatoes, bell pepper, onion, couscous, and chickpea mixture. Add the tahini sauce and mix well. Divide among 4 storage containers.

- **Storage:** Store in the refrigerator for up to 5 days. Serve cold.

- **Gluten-free option:** Use quinoa instead of couscous.

- **Vegan option:** Use agave instead of honey.

Per Serving: Calories: 655; Total fat: 24g; Carbohydrates: 87g; Fiber: 18g; Protein: 24g; Calcium: 184mg; Vitamin D: 0 IU; Potassium: 906mg; Magnesium: 116mg; Sodium: 73mg

ROASTED EGGPLANT SANDWICHES

Makes 2 sandwiches
Prep time: 10 minutes • **Cook time:** 30 minutes
EGG-FREE • NUT-FREE

When cooked, eggplant takes on a tender texture and savory flavor. It can be a handy alternative to your favorite meats. Eggplant is also a superfood, offering few calories but a great deal of fiber and antioxidants. These essential nutrients help regulate your blood sugar, reduce your risk of heart disease, and may even aid in weight loss. A lot of benefit from a little plant.

Nonstick cooking spray (optional)
1 small eggplant, cut crosswise into
⅓-inch-thick slices
1 tablespoon extra-virgin olive oil
¼ teaspoon freshly ground black pepper

1 tomato, sliced
1 small red onion, sliced
½ cup chopped fresh basil
4 ounces fresh burrata cheese
4 whole wheat bread slices

1. Preheat the oven to 375°F. Line a sheet pan with aluminum foil or coat with nonstick cooking spray.
2. Brush both sides of the eggplant with the oil, put on the prepared sheet pan, and season with the pepper. Roast for about 25 minutes, or until the skin is wrinkly and the eggplant is soft and let cool.
3. Divide the roasted eggplant into 2 portions and place in one partition of 2 divided storage containers. Divide the tomato, onion, and basil into the second partition. Store the burrata cheese and bread in their own separate containers.
4. To serve, reheat the eggplant in the microwave for 30 seconds to 1 minute. For each sandwich, toast 2 bread slices. Layer one-quarter of the cheese on a slice of toast and top with the eggplant, tomato, and onion. Add the basil and close the sandwich.

- **Storage:** Store all the sandwich components in the refrigerator for up to 5 days.

- **Variations:** Instead of basil, use arugula dressed with a little lemon juice, and use Parmesan cheese instead of burrata to add a little bit of earthiness and tang.

Per Serving (1 sandwich): Calories: 542; Total fat: 24g; Carbohydrates: 56g; Fiber: 9g; Protein: 21g; Calcium: 469mg; Vitamin D: 0 IU; Potassium: 524mg; Magnesium: 35mg; Sodium: 308mg

BLACK BEAN BURGERS

Makes 4 burgers
Prep time: 15 minutes • **Cook time:** 20 minutes
DAIRY-FREE • NUT-FREE

These delicious, protein-rich patties are also full of fiber, which will help you stay satisfied longer. Top them like you would any other burger. They pair nicely with the Summer Rainbow Pasta Salad (page 112) and the Sweet Potatoes with Chopped Pistachios (page 113).

Nonstick cooking spray
2 tablespoons extra-virgin olive oil, divided
½ large green bell pepper, coarsely chopped
½ small onion, coarsely chopped
3 garlic cloves, peeled
1 large egg
1 tablespoon ground cumin

½ teaspoon garlic powder
¼ teaspoon paprika
1 teaspoon freshly ground black pepper
½ teaspoon salt
½ cup dried unseasoned bread crumbs
1 (15-ounce) can no-salt-added black beans, drained and rinsed

1. Preheat the oven to 375°F. Coat a sheet pan with cooking spray.
2. In a large skillet, heat 1 tablespoon of oil over medium heat. Add the bell pepper, onion, and garlic and sauté until softened.
3. In a small bowl, whisk together the egg, remaining 1 tablespoon of oil, the cumin, garlic powder, paprika, black pepper, and salt until well combined.
4. In a food processor, combine the sautéed vegetables, bread crumbs, and egg mixture and pulse everything together. Add the black beans and pulse, leaving some bigger chunks of beans.
5. Divide the mixture into 4 portions and form into patties. Put the patties on the prepared sheet pan and bake for 10 minutes on each side. Divide into 4 storage containers.

• **Storage:** Store in the refrigerator for up to 5 days or in the freezer for up to 3 months. To reheat, vent the lid slightly, and microwave on medium for 60 to 90 seconds. To reheat from frozen, microwave on medium for 2 to 3 minutes.

Per Serving (1 burger): Calories: 292; Total fat: 17g; Carbohydrates: 29g; Fiber: 6.5g; Protein: 10g; Calcium: 100mg; Vitamin D: 10 IU; Potassium: 326mg; Magnesium: 58mg; Sodium: 403mg

TOFU STIR-FRY

Serves 4

Prep time: 10 minutes • **Cook time:** 15 minutes

DAIRY-FREE • EGG-FREE • NUT-FREE • VEGAN OPTION (SEE TIP)

Legend has it that tofu was discovered 2,000 years ago when a Chinese cook accidentally curdled soy milk by adding seaweed. If you are a newbie to cooking tofu, this delicious, quick stir-fry is the perfect way to start. The combination of textures—from the crunchy vegetables to flavors from the honey and soy sauce—allows the tofu to mix in, providing a gentle introduction of this protein-packed food.

---

1 tablespoon canola oil

2 large garlic cloves, minced

2½ tablespoons reduced-sodium soy sauce, divided

1 tablespoon minced fresh ginger

1 small bunch scallions, finely chopped, divided

1 cup sugar snap peas

1 cup small broccoli florets

½ cup diced carrots

½ cup sliced red bell pepper

1 tablespoon honey

10 ounces spinach leaves, divided

2 (14-ounce) packages extra-firm tofu, drained, patted dry, and cut into ¾-inch cubes

1. In a large wok, sauté pan, or deep skillet, heat the oil over medium heat and swirl to coat the entire pan. Once hot, add the garlic, 1 tablespoon of soy sauce, and the ginger. Stir well for about a minute. Add the scallions, snap peas, broccoli, carrots, and bell pepper and stir-fry for 5 to 8 minutes, or until the vegetables are crisp-tender.

2. Add the remaining 1½ tablespoons of soy sauce and the honey. Add 5 ounces of spinach, making sure to stir as it cooks down. Once it has wilted, add the remaining 5 ounces of spinach. Stir until it has cooked down. Add the tofu and continue stirring occasionally for 2 to 3 minutes to give the tofu time to absorb the flavors. Divide into 4 storage containers.

- **Storage:** Store in the refrigerator for up to 5 days or in the freezer for up to 3 months. Reheat in the microwave for about 90 seconds. To reheat from frozen, microwave on medium for 3 to 4 minutes.

- **Vegan option:** Use agave instead of honey.

  Per Serving: Calories: 304; Total fat: 14g; Carbohydrates: 21g; Fiber: 7g; Protein: 25g; Calcium: 277mg; Vitamin D: 0 IU; Potassium: 658mg; Magnesium: 72mg; Sodium: 445mg

SPINACH AND MUSHROOM LASAGNA

Serves 10
Prep time: 20 minutes • **Cook time:** 55 minutes
NUT-FREE • VEGETARIAN

This lasagna is so rich in flavor and texture you won't even miss the meat. Comforting and filling, it also provides you with a combination of antioxidants, fiber, and calcium—all heart-healthy nutrients that are DASH essentials. This is a great recipe to make a double batch and store in the freezer for a busy week later on.

12 whole wheat lasagna noodles

1½ pounds cremini mushrooms, coarsely chopped

1 medium zucchini, cut into ½-inch pieces

1 medium yellow squash, cut into ½-inch pieces

2 tablespoons extra-virgin olive oil

1 large onion, chopped

4 garlic cloves, minced

3 cups spinach leaves

1 cup no-salt-added tomato sauce

1 (6-ounce) can no-salt-added tomato paste

1 (28-ounce) can no-salt-added crushed tomatoes

½ teaspoon salt

1 teaspoon freshly ground black pepper

3 large eggs, beaten

1 (15-ounce) container 1% cottage cheese

4 cups shredded part-skim low-moisture mozzarella cheese, divided

¾ cup grated Parmesan cheese, divided

1 tablespoon dried basil

1 teaspoon garlic powder

1 teaspoon onion powder

1. Preheat the oven to 350°F.
2. Bring a large pot of water to a boil. Add the lasagna noodles and cook until al dente according to the package directions. Drain and lay them flat on a sheet of aluminum foil.
3. In a large sauté pan or deep skillet, dry-sauté the mushrooms over medium heat until moisture starts releasing. Then add the zucchini and squash. When the mushrooms are no longer releasing moisture, add the oil, onion, garlic, and spinach. Sauté, stirring frequently, for 2 to 3 minutes, or until all the vegetables have softened. Add the tomato sauce, tomato paste, and crushed tomatoes and stir in the salt and pepper.
4. In a large bowl, mix together the eggs, cottage cheese, 2½ cups of mozzarella cheese, ½ cup of Parmesan cheese, the basil, garlic powder, and onion powder.

Continued ❯

5. In a 9-by-13-inch baking dish, spread some of the tomato and vegetable sauce mixture to cover the bottom. Make 3 layers in this order: 3 lasagna noodles, one-third of the cheese and egg mixture, one-third of the remaining tomato sauce. Top with a final layer of noodles and the remaining 1 ½ cups of mozzarella and ¼ cup of Parmesan cheeses.

6. Cover with foil and bake for 40 minutes. Remove the foil and bake for an additional 10 to 15 minutes, or until browned and bubbling. Let cool completely before cutting into 10 portions. Place a portion in each of 10 containers.

- **Storage:** Store in the refrigerator for up to 5 days or in the freezer for up to 3 months. To reheat, vent the lid slightly, and microwave on medium for 2 minutes. To reheat from the freezer, thaw overnight in the refrigerator, and follow the refrigerated instructions.

- **Cooking tip:** To make this recipe a little quicker, you can use no-boil noodles and jarred no-salt-added spaghetti sauce instead of crushed tomatoes, paste, and sauce.

Per Serving: Calories: 438; Total fat: 17g; Carbohydrates: 44g; Fiber: 7.5g; Protein: 28g; Calcium: 382mg; Vitamin D: 23 IU; Potassium: 1,126mg; Magnesium: 101mg; Sodium: 782mg

MUSHROOM BOLOGNESE

Serves 4
Prep time: 10 minutes • **Cook time:** 25 minutes
EGG-FREE • NUT-FREE

Here is a meat-heavy classic given a DASH-friendly makeover. It is still filled with umami tastes and satisfying textures, but the special bonus is in its dose of fiber. Fiber helps us feel full and has both digestive and heart health benefits.

8 ounces whole wheat penne pasta

2 tablespoons extra-virgin olive oil

1 small onion, diced

1 large carrot, diced

2 celery stalks, diced

4 garlic cloves, minced

1 pound mushrooms, diced

⅔ cup dry red wine

1 bay leaf

2 cups low-sodium vegetable broth

1 (15-ounce) can no-salt-added tomato sauce

1 teaspoon Italian seasoning

¼ teaspoon freshly ground black pepper

¼ teaspoon red pepper flakes (optional)

½ cup grated Parmesan cheese

1. Bring a large pot of water to a boil. Add the pasta and cook until al dente according to the package directions. Drain well.
2. Meanwhile, in a large sauté pan or deep skillet, heat the oil over medium-high heat. Add the onion, carrot, and celery and cook for 5 to 7 minutes, or until the vegetables are soft and the onion is translucent. Add the garlic and mushrooms and cook for 4 to 5 minutes, or until the mushrooms are browned.
3. Stir in the wine, add the bay leaf, bring to a boil, and cook for 2 to 3 minutes, or until the wine is reduced by half. Remove the bay leaf. Add the vegetable broth, tomato sauce, Italian seasoning, black pepper, and red pepper flakes (if using).
4. In a large bowl, toss the drained pasta with the sauce. Divide into 4 storage containers and top each serving with 2 tablespoons of Parmesan cheese.

- **Storage:** Store in the refrigerator for up to 5 days or in the freezer for up to 3 months. Reheat by microwaving on medium for 90 seconds. If frozen, reheat in the microwave on medium for 3 minutes. Adding a splash of water, milk, or broth helps foods maintain their moisture.

Per Serving: Calories: 456; Total fat: 12g; Carbohydrates: 70g; Fiber: 10g; Protein: 18g; Calcium: 149mg; Vitamin D: 5 IU; Potassium: 819mg; Magnesium: 104mg; Sodium: 344mg

FIVE-BEAN CHILI

Serves 6
Prep time: 10 minutes • **Cook time:** 30 minutes
DAIRY-FREE • EGG-FREE • GLUTEN-FREE • NUT-FREE • VEGAN

This chili is the perfect weeknight dish—it's quick, easy, and reheats well. The focus here is on getting something satisfying with a little bit of flavor. You'll get protein, fiber, and essential vitamins and minerals from the beans. With the cumin and chili seasoning, you'll get a nice smoky taste and a little bit of heat.

2 tablespoons extra-virgin olive oil

1 medium onion, diced

1 green bell pepper, diced

2 garlic cloves, minced

1 (28-ounce) can no-salt-added crushed tomatoes

1 tablespoon chili powder

1 teaspoon ground cumin

1 (15-ounce) can no-salt-added black beans, drained and rinsed

1 (15-ounce) can no-salt-added pinto beans, drained and rinsed

1 (15-ounce) can no-salt-added kidney beans, drained and rinsed

1 (15-ounce) can no-salt-added navy beans, drained and rinsed

1 (15-ounce) can no-salt-added chickpeas, drained and rinsed

10 scallions, chopped

1. In a large pot, heat the oil over medium-high heat. Add the onion and bell pepper and cook for 5 to 7 minutes, or until the onion is translucent.
2. Add the garlic and cook for 1 minute. Stir in the crushed tomatoes, chili powder, cumin, black beans, pinto beans, kidney beans, navy beans, and chickpeas. Reduce the heat to a simmer and cook, stirring frequently, for 20 minutes to thicken slightly and blend the flavors. Divide among 6 storage containers. Store the scallions separately. Top the chili with the scallions after reheating to serve.

- **Storage:** Store in the refrigerator for up to 5 days or in the freezer for up to 3 months. Reheat for 1 to 2 minutes in the microwave, stirring once. To reheat from the freezer, microwave on medium for 4 to 5 minutes.

Per Serving: Calories: 425; Total fat: 6.5g; Carbohydrates: 67g; Fiber: 23g; Protein: 23g; Calcium: 256mg; Vitamin D: 0 IU; Potassium: 1,431mg; Magnesium: 184mg; Sodium: 58mg

SPINACH, KALE, AND CHEESE CRÊPES

Makes 8 crêpes
Prep time: 10 minutes • **Cook time:** 20 minutes
NUT-FREE • VEGETARIAN • GLUTEN-FREE OPTION (SEE TIP)

It's never a bad time to get more creative with your green leafy vegetables. Here, we take kale and spinach and sauté them with garlic and herbs. This gives them a lot of flavor on top of their already great nutritional value. Green leafy vegetables are powerhouses, offering essential minerals like iron, calcium, potassium, and magnesium. They're also a great source of vitamins, including vitamins C, E, K, and many B vitamins.

Nonstick cooking spray

1 cup whole wheat flour

2 large eggs

½ cup 1% milk

½ cup water

¼ teaspoon salt

2 teaspoons extra-virgin olive oil, divided

1 garlic clove, minced

1 cup chopped spinach

1 cup chopped kale leaves

1 cup chopped fresh parsley

1 tablespoon fresh thyme

¼ teaspoon freshly ground black pepper

¼ cup shredded part-skim low-moisture mozzarella cheese

1. Preheat the broiler to 500°F. Coat a 9-by-13-inch broiler-safe baking dish with cooking spray.
2. In a large bowl, whisk together the flour and eggs. Gradually add the milk, water, and salt, stirring until well combined.
3. Grease a nonstick skillet with 1 teaspoon of oil and heat over medium-high heat. Pour ¼ cup of the batter into the skillet. Tilt the skillet in a circular motion so the batter coats the surface evenly. Cook the crêpe for about 2 minutes, or until the bottom is lightly browned. Repeat to make a total of 8 crêpes.
4. In a separate skillet, heat the remaining 1 teaspoon of oil over medium heat. Add the garlic and cook, stirring rapidly, for 30 seconds. Add the spinach, kale, parsley, thyme, and pepper. Cook, stirring occasionally, for 3 to 5 minutes, or until the spinach and kale have wilted.

Continued ❯

5. Divide the spinach mixture and mozzarella cheese evenly among the crêpes. Roll up the crêpes and place in the prepared baking dish. Set under the broiler for a few minutes, just to melt the cheese, keeping a close eye on it. Divide the crêpes among 4 storage containers.

- **Storage:** Store in the refrigerator for up to 5 days. To reheat, microwave on medium for 90 seconds.

- **Gluten-free option:** Use all-purpose gluten-free flour.

  Per Serving (2 crêpes): Calories: 253; Total fat: 15g; Carbohydrates: 26g; Fiber: 4g; Protein: 11g; Calcium: 137mg; Vitamin D: 36 IU; Potassium: 349mg; Magnesium: 66mg; Sodium: 255mg

GARDEN VEGETABLE AND CHEESE QUICHE

Serves 8
Prep time: 20 minutes • **Cook time:** 55 minutes
NUT-FREE • VEGETARIAN

Getting a hefty dose of vegetables is far easier when served in a tasty quiche. This veggie-loaded quiche is a fiber, vitamin, and antioxidant powerhouse. Enjoy this meal for breakfast, lunch, or dinner. Pair it with Tomato-Basil Soup (page 123) or Kale-Poppy Seed Salad (page 119).

1 (9-inch) unbaked deep-dish piecrust

1 tablespoon extra-virgin olive oil

½ medium red onion, finely chopped

1 large green bell pepper, chopped

½ cup sliced cremini mushrooms

1 small zucchini, chopped

1 large tomato, chopped

6 large eggs

½ cup 1% milk

2 tablespoons all-purpose flour

2 teaspoons dried basil

½ teaspoon salt

½ teaspoon freshly ground black pepper

1½ cups shredded Monterey Jack
   cheese, divided

1. Preheat the oven to 350°F.
2. Bake the crust for 7 to 8 minutes to set. Remove from the oven, but leave the oven on.
3. In a large skillet, heat the oil over medium heat. Add the onion and sauté for about 1 minute. Add the bell pepper, mushrooms, zucchini, and tomato and cook for 5 to 7 minutes, or until soft. Remove from the heat and set aside.
4. In a medium bowl, whisk together the eggs, milk, flour, basil, salt, and black pepper. Stir in 1 cup of Monterey Jack cheese. Pour the mixture into the baked piecrust. Top with the remaining ½ cup of cheese.
5. Bake for 40 to 50 minutes, or until the mixture is cooked through. Cool for 10 minutes before cutting into 8 wedges. Divide the wedges among 8 storage containers.

- **Storage:** Store in the refrigerator for up to 5 days. To reheat, vent the lid slightly, and microwave on medium for 90 seconds.

  Per Serving: Calories: 266; Total fat: 17g; Carbohydrates: 17g; Fiber: 1g; Protein: 12g; Calcium: 209mg; Vitamin D: 43 IU; Potassium: 259mg; Magnesium: 21mg; Sodium: 422mg

RIGATONI WITH SPINACH PESTO

Serves 4
Prep time: 15 minutes • **Cook time:** 25 minutes
EGG-FREE • VEGETARIAN

Who doesn't love a good pesto? Here, we swap out the traditional basil for spinach, which is an excellent source of iron and calcium. The whole grains in the pasta add a bit of protein and provide fiber, aiding in digestion and heart health. If you want, you can just make the pesto, because in addition to being great on pasta, it also works well as a vegetable dip or salad dressing. You can freeze the pesto for up to 3 months.

FOR THE SPINACH PESTO

4 cups baby spinach

½ cup walnuts or pine nuts

4 garlic cloves, peeled

¼ cup grated Parmesan cheese

½ teaspoon freshly ground black pepper

1 teaspoon fresh lemon juice

½ cup extra-virgin olive oil

FOR THE RIGATONI

8 ounces whole wheat rigatoni pasta

Nonstick cooking spray

1 cup shredded part-skim low-moisture
   mozzarella cheese

1 tablespoon chopped fresh basil

TO MAKE THE SPINACH PESTO

1. In a food processor, pulse together the spinach, nuts, garlic, Parmesan cheese, pepper, and lemon juice. With the machine running, stream in the oil and blend until the nuts are very fine.

TO MAKE THE RIGATONI

2. Bring a large pot of water to a boil. Add the pasta and cook until al dente according to the package directions. Drain well.

3. Preheat the oven to 350°F. Coat a 7-by-11-inch baking dish with nonstick cooking spray.

4. In a large bowl, toss the cooked pasta with the pesto. Pour into the prepared baking dish and sprinkle with the mozzarella cheese.

5. Cover with foil or a lid and bake for 20 minutes. Uncover and bake for another 15 minutes to melt the cheese.
6. Sprinkle with the basil. Let stand for 5 minutes before portioning into 4 storage containers.

- **Storage:** Store in the refrigerator for up to 5 days or in the freezer for up to 2 months. To thaw, place in the refrigerator overnight. To reheat, vent the lid, and microwave for 2 minutes.

- **Variations:** If you want a nonvegetarian version, add cooked diced or shredded chicken when tossing the pasta with pesto before baking.

  Per Serving: Calories: 648; Total fat: 47g; Carbohydrates: 47g; Fiber: 7.5g; Protein: 18g; Calcium: 231mg; Vitamin D: 4 IU; Potassium: 341mg; Magnesium: 139mg; Sodium: 224mg

Crab and Sweet Potato Cakes
Page 157

CHAPTER 7

Fish & Shellfish

SHRIMP CEVICHE

Serves 4
Prep time: 30 minutes, plus 30 minutes to marinate • **Cook time:** 10 minutes
DAIRY-FREE • EGG-FREE • GLUTEN-FREE • NUT-FREE

Having grown up on the coast of Ecuador, Maria-Paula considers ceviche a comfort food. Light yet flavorful, this is a dish that can be served almost any time of day, either as an appetizer or a main course. Add some popcorn to this for additional crunch; tortilla chips also work great.

2 pounds medium shrimp, peeled, deveined, and cooked
¾ cup fresh lime juice
¼ cup fresh lemon juice
⅓ cup fresh orange juice
1 cup finely chopped red onion

¾ cup diced cucumber
2 small roma (plum) tomatoes, seeded and diced
1 cup chopped fresh cilantro
1 avocado, pitted, peeled, and chopped

1. In a large bowl, combine the shrimp, lime juice, lemon juice, and orange juice. Cover and refrigerate for 30 minutes.
2. Add the onion, cucumber, tomatoes, cilantro, and avocado to the bowl. Toss to coat and mix evenly. Divide into 4 storage containers.

- **Storage:** Store in the refrigerator for up to 5 days. To avoid browned avocados, consider adding them right before serving or using frozen avocado chunks thawed in the refrigerator the morning of, so they will be ready by mealtime.

- **Variations:** Swap out the shrimp for raw fish—bass, snapper, or halibut are best. Double the citrus juices and cover the fish with it. Marinate in the refrigerator for at least 4 hours.

  Per Serving: Calories: 259; Total fat: 6.5g; Carbohydrates: 11g; Fiber: 3.5g; Protein: 41g; Calcium: 151mg; Vitamin D: 0 IU; Potassium: 919mg; Magnesium: 93mg; Sodium: 243mg

PINEAPPLE AND SHRIMP SKEWERS

Makes 8 skewers
Prep time: 15 minutes, plus soaking time for skewers • **Cook time:** 25 minutes
DAIRY-FREE • EGG-FREE • NUT-FREE

These grilled skewers are sweet and light—perfect for a summer barbecue or backyard party. Grilled pineapple is such a fun way to add a spin to any kebab recipe. Here, we pair it with shrimp, a rich source of omega-3 fatty acids, which helps promote heart and brain health. If you don't have a grill, don't fret. See the cooking tip on page 150 for alternate instructions.

¼ cup honey

Juice of ½ medium orange

Juice of 2 limes

1 tablespoon extra-virgin olive oil

2 teaspoons reduced-sodium soy sauce

1 teaspoon freshly ground black pepper

¼ teaspoon chili powder

1 small green bell pepper, cut into
  1-inch squares

1 small red bell pepper, cut into 1-inch squares

1 small red onion, cut into 1-inch chunks

1 pound peeled and deveined shrimp (32 to 40),
  fresh or (thawed) frozen

2 cups cubed (1-inch) pineapple

1. If using wooden skewers, soak them in water for 30 to 60 minutes before grilling. Preheat the grill to medium heat (350°F to 400°F).
2. In a small bowl, whisk together the honey, orange juice, lime juice, oil, soy sauce, black pepper, and chili powder until well mixed. Set aside.
3. Assemble 8 skewers by alternating ingredients: a veggie chunk, a shrimp, a veggie chunk, a pineapple chunk, and another veggie chunk (such as: green bell pepper, a shrimp, an onion chunk, a pineapple chunk, and a red bell pepper), repeating until there is about 1 inch left at the bottom of the skewer and ½ inch at the top. Brush the skewers all over with the honey and soy sauce marinade until all sides are fully coated. Let them rest for at least 10 minutes.
4. Put the skewers on the grill and cook, flipping once, for 4 to 5 minutes per side, or until the shrimp are cooked through. While grilling, brush the skewers with more marinade. Place 2 skewers in each of 4 storage containers.

Continued ❯

- **Storage:** Store in the refrigerator for up to 5 days or in the freezer for up to 2 months. To reheat, vent the lid slightly, and microwave on medium for 2 minutes. If reheating from frozen, microwave on medium for 3 minutes.

- **Cooking tip:** If you don't have a grill, broil the kebabs on a sheet pan for 2 minutes on each side.

  Per Serving (2 skewers): Calories: 260; Total fat: 4g; Carbohydrates: 35g; Fiber: 2.5g; Protein: 24g; Calcium: 96mg; Vitamin D: 0 IU; Potassium: 554mg; Magnesium: 60mg; Sodium: 235mg

LEMON-DILL TILAPIA

Serves 4

Prep time: 5 minutes • **Cook time:** 20 minutes

EGG-FREE • GLUTEN-FREE • NUT-FREE • DAIRY-FREE OPTION (SEE TIP)

Simple yet delicious, mild tilapia—inexpensive, widely available, and a great source of omega-3 fatty acids—is bathed in a buttery lemon-dill sauce. Pair this dish with Mashed Sweet Potatoes (page 111) and Crisp and Sweet Quinoa (page 107).

4 (4-ounce) tilapia fillets

¼ teaspoon salt

½ teaspoon freshly ground black pepper

2 tablespoons unsalted butter

2 large lemons, 1 juiced, 1 sliced

¼ cup chopped fresh dill

1. Preheat the oven to 350°F.
2. Put the tilapia fillets in a glass baking dish. Season with the salt and pepper.
3. Top each fillet with ½ tablespoon of butter, the lemon juice, and 1 tablespoon of dill. Once they are coated, place the lemon slices on top.
4. Bake for 15 to 20 minutes, or until the fish flakes with a fork. Divide among 4 storage containers.

- **Storage:** Store in the refrigerator for up to 5 days or in the freezer for up to 3 months. To reheat, vent the lid slightly, and microwave on medium for 90 seconds. If reheating from frozen, microwave on medium for 3 minutes.

- **Dairy-free option:** Use extra-virgin olive oil instead of butter.

Per Serving: Calories: 163; Total fat: 8g; Carbohydrates: 1g; Fiber: 0g; Protein: 22g; Calcium: 17mg; Vitamin D: 128 IU; Potassium: 345mg; Magnesium: 31mg; Sodium: 194mg

SESAME-CRUSTED AHI TUNA STEAKS

Serves 4
Prep time: 5 minutes • **Cook time:** 4 to 6 minutes
DAIRY-FREE • EGG-FREE • NUT-FREE

Seeds pack a ton of nutrition for their relatively small size. Sesame seeds, for instance, are rich in B vitamins and a host of minerals, such as iron, magnesium, calcium, phosphorus, and zinc. Here, we add both black and white sesame seeds to the tuna for visual interest and extra flavor.

2 tablespoons reduced-sodium soy sauce
1 tablespoon sesame oil
1 tablespoon rice vinegar
½ tablespoon honey
4 (4-ounce) ahi tuna steaks

¼ cup white sesame seeds
¼ cup black sesame seeds
1 tablespoon extra-virgin olive oil
2 scallions, chopped

1. In a small bowl, mix together the soy sauce, sesame oil, vinegar, and honey.
2. Coat the tuna steaks with the mixture.
3. Spread the white and black sesame seeds out on a plate and press both sides of each tuna steak into the seeds to coat.
4. In a skillet or nonstick pan, heat the olive oil over high heat. Sear the tuna steaks for 30 to 45 seconds on each side. You'll know the tuna is done when it has been seared white on the outside but remains pink in the middle. Divide among 4 storage containers. Top with the scallions.

- **Storage:** Store in the refrigerator for up to 5 days or in the freezer for up to 4 months. Thaw in the refrigerator overnight. Serve cold or sauté with a little olive oil in a skillet until warm.

- **Ingredient tip:** Raw fish can potentially harbor harmful bacteria or parasites, so when cooking fish to medium-rare as in this dish, the FDA recommends freezing it for 7 days before cooking. Thaw overnight in the refrigerator.

Per Serving: Calories: 302; Total fat: 17g; Carbohydrates: 6g; Fiber: 1.5g; Protein: 32g; Calcium: 110mg; Vitamin D: 77 IU; Potassium: 627mg; Magnesium: 78mg; Sodium: 345mg

GRILLED HALIBUT WITH BLACK BEAN AND MANGO SALSA

Serves 4

Prep time: 15 minutes • **Cook time:** 10 minutes

DAIRY-FREE • EGG-FREE • GLUTEN-FREE • NUT-FREE

Halibut provides a handful of heart-healthy nutrients, like omega-3 fatty acids, phosphorus, and magnesium. Paired with this versatile salsa, the dish packs a colorful and flavorful punch. No grill? No problem. See the cooking tip for alternate instructions.

---

1 (15-ounce) can no-salt-added black beans, drained and rinsed

1 (15-ounce) can juice-packed diced mango, drained

½ medium red onion, chopped

½ medium red bell pepper, diced

3 tablespoons minced fresh cilantro

Juice of 1 large lime

Juice of 1 large lemon

3 tablespoons extra-virgin olive oil

1 teaspoon freshly ground black pepper

1 garlic clove, minced

4 (4-ounce) halibut fillets

1. Preheat the grill to medium-high heat (350°F to 400°F). In a large bowl, mix together the beans, mango, onion, bell pepper, cilantro, and lime juice. Divide into 4 storage containers.
2. In a small bowl, mix together the lemon juice, oil, black pepper, and garlic.
3. Coat the halibut fillets in the lemon marinade and let rest for 10 minutes.
4. Grill for 2 minutes on each side. Take off the grill and allow it to rest. Divide into 4 storage containers.
5. To serve, reheat and top each fillet with a generous serving of the salsa.

- **Storage:** Store in the refrigerator for up to 5 days or in the freezer for up to 2 months. To reheat the fish, vent the lid slightly, and microwave on medium for 90 seconds. If frozen, thaw in the refrigerator overnight, and microwave before serving. Top with the salsa before serving.

- **Cooking tip:** To bake the halibut, preheat the oven to 400°F. Coat a sheet pan with cooking spray. Bake for 5 to 6 minutes on each side.

Per Serving: Calories: 340; Total fat: 13g; Carbohydrates: 31g; Fiber: 6g; Protein: 26g; Calcium: 71mg; Vitamin D: 196 IU; Potassium: 779mg; Magnesium: 81mg; Sodium: 94mg

JERK SALMON

Serves 4

Prep time: 5 minutes • **Cook time:** 12 to 15 minutes

DAIRY-FREE • EGG-FREE • GLUTEN-FREE • NUT-FREE

Cooking with less salt can be a challenge for some people as they start the DASH diet, but building your pantry with other herbs and spices makes it a lot easier. One versatile spice rub that helps add flavor at home is jerk seasoning, which originated in Jamaica and involves thyme, allspice, cinnamon, and cayenne pepper. It's great on salmon and can be used on many other fish, along with meats like chicken, pork, and beef.

2 tablespoons extra-virgin olive oil, divided

2½ teaspoons dried thyme

2 teaspoons ground allspice

2 teaspoons onion powder

2 teaspoons freshly ground black pepper

½ teaspoon ground cinnamon

½ teaspoon cayenne pepper

4 (4-ounce) skin-on salmon fillets

1. Preheat the oven to 350°F. Lightly coat a sheet pan with ½ tablespoon of oil.
2. In a small bowl, mix together the thyme, allspice, onion powder, black pepper, cinnamon, and cayenne pepper. Lightly coat the salmon fillets with the remaining 1½ tablespoons of oil and season with the rub.
3. Place the salmon, skin-side down, on the prepared sheet pan. Bake for 12 to 15 minutes, or until the salmon is cooked through and flakes easily with a fork. Divide among 4 storage containers.

- **Storage:** Store in the refrigerator for up to 5 days or in the freezer for up to 3 months. Salmon may be eaten cold or hot. Reheat for 90 seconds in the microwave. To reheat from the freezer, microwave on medium for about 3 minutes.

Per Serving: Calories: 255; Total fat: 15g; Carbohydrates: 3g; Fiber: 1g; Protein: 26g; Calcium: 46mg; Vitamin D: 283 IU; Potassium: 677mg; Magnesium: 44mg; Sodium: 59mg

MEDITERRANEAN-HERBED SCALLOPS

Serves 4
Prep time: 5 minutes • **Cook time:** 12 to 15 minutes
DAIRY-FREE • EGG-FREE • GLUTEN-FREE • NUT-FREE

Because scallops have a mild taste, they pair well with many different herbs and spices. Here, we boost the flavor profile with fresh rosemary, sage, basil, and thyme. Scallops are an excellent source of several trace minerals, including the antioxidant selenium, and they provide essential omega-3 fatty acids.

¼ cup fresh basil leaves

¼ cup fresh thyme leaves

1 tablespoon fresh rosemary leaves

1 tablespoon chopped fresh sage

2 teaspoons freshly ground black pepper

1 tablespoon fresh lemon juice

3 tablespoons extra-virgin olive oil, divided

1 garlic clove, minced

12 scallops

4 lemon wedges (optional)

1. In a food processor or blender, combine the basil, thyme, rosemary, sage, pepper, lemon juice, and 1½ tablespoons of oil. Pulse until mixed. The herbs should still be visible.
2. In a large skillet, heat the remaining 1½ tablespoons of oil over medium-high heat. Add the garlic and cook, stirring rapidly, for 30 seconds. Working in batches, sear the scallops on each side, for 2 to 3 minutes per side. Remove from the skillet and top with the herbed oil. Place 3 herb-topped scallops in each of 4 storage containers.
3. To serve, after reheating the scallops, place a lemon wedge on the side (if using).

• **Storage:** Store in the refrigerator for up to 5 days or in the freezer for up to 3 months. Thaw in the refrigerator overnight. To reheat, bake at 325°F for up to 10 minutes, or sauté with a little olive oil in a skillet until warm.

• **Variations:** Feel free to change the protein here; this recipe also works well with mild white fish, chicken, or pork.

Per Serving: Calories: 158; Total fat: 11g; Carbohydrates: 5g; Fiber: 1g; Protein: 11g; Calcium: 39mg; Vitamin D: 1 IU; Potassium: 223mg; Magnesium: 29mg; Sodium: 335mg

PISTACHIO-CRUSTED TILAPIA

Serves 4
Prep time: 10 minutes • **Cook time:** 15 minutes
EGG-FREE • NUT-FREE OPTION (SEE TIP)

Fast and easy, this fish entrée is a popular weeknight option. The mixture of bread crumbs and pistachios gives the fish an added crunch and an amazing mouthfeel. Squeeze some lemon or orange juice over the fish before serving for a citrus twist.

Nonstick cooking spray

4 (4-ounce) tilapia fillets

¼ teaspoon salt

½ teaspoon freshly ground black pepper

½ teaspoon garlic powder

¼ cup nonfat plain Greek yogurt

½ cup dried unseasoned bread crumbs

½ cup raw pistachios, finely chopped

1 teaspoon dried oregano

1 teaspoon dried thyme

1. Preheat the oven to 375°F. Cover a sheet pan with foil and coat with nonstick cooking spray.
2. Season the fillets with the salt, pepper, and garlic powder. Spread 1 tablespoon of yogurt onto each fillet until evenly coated. Set aside.
3. In a shallow dish, mix together the bread crumbs, pistachios, oregano, and thyme.
4. Press each fillet in the pistachio and bread crumb mixture on both sides until well coated.
5. Arrange the fillets on the prepared sheet pan and bake for 12 to 15 minutes, or until cooked through. Divide among 4 storage containers.

- **Storage:** Store in the refrigerator for up to 5 days or in the freezer for 3 to 4 months. To reheat, vent the lid slightly, and microwave on medium for 90 seconds. To reheat from the freezer, microwave on medium for about 3 minutes.

- **Nut-free option:** Use hulled pumpkin seeds or sunflower seeds instead of pistachios in the same quantity.

  Per Serving: Calories: 348; Total fat: 21g; Carbohydrates: 16g; Fiber: 2.5g; Protein: 29g; Calcium: 86mg; Vitamin D: 128 IU; Potassium: 520mg; Magnesium: 50mg; Sodium: 348mg

CRAB AND SWEET POTATO CAKES

Serves 4
Prep time: 15 minutes, plus 30 minutes to chill • **Cook time:** 40 minutes
NUT-FREE

Crab cakes are a tasty, filling dish, but here they get a DASH makeover. By replacing the usual fat-heavy ingredients with fresh herbs, a little bit of citrus, and a little bit of sweetness from the sweet potatoes, this dish gives you fewer calories, more fiber, and essential vitamins and minerals. We've worked to maintain a nice crunch with the bread crumbs, a must for the perfect crab cake.

FOR THE SAUCE

⅔ cup nonfat plain Greek yogurt

2 tablespoons chopped fresh parsley

2 tablespoons chopped fresh basil

2 tablespoons fresh lemon juice

1 garlic clove, minced

FOR THE CRAB CAKES

2 large sweet potatoes, peeled and halved

1 tablespoon nonfat plain Greek yogurt

¼ teaspoon freshly ground black pepper

¼ teaspoon dried thyme

¼ cup chopped fresh parsley

¼ cup chopped red onion

1 pound lump crabmeat

½ cup dried unseasoned bread crumbs

1 large egg

2 tablespoons extra-virgin olive oil, divided

4 lemon wedges (optional)

TO MAKE THE SAUCE

1. In a small bowl, mix together the yogurt, parsley, basil, lemon juice, and garlic until well combined. Divide the sauce among 4 small storage containers.

TO MAKE THE CRAB CAKES

2. Bring a medium pot of water to a boil. Add the sweet potatoes and cook for 15 to 20 minutes, or until soft. Transfer to a bowl and let cool.

3. Smash the sweet potatoes. Add the yogurt, pepper, thyme, parsley, and onion and mix well. Add the crabmeat and bread crumbs and mix. Finally, add the egg and mix well.

4. Gently form into 8 cakes and set on a plate. Refrigerate for 30 minutes to set nicely.

Continued ❯

5. In a cast-iron or nonstick skillet, heat 1 tablespoon of oil over medium heat. Add 4 crab cakes, and cook, turning once, for about 8 minutes total, or until browned on each side. Repeat with the remaining crab cakes and 1 tablespoon of oil. Place 2 crab cakes in each of 4 storage containers.

6. When ready to serve, reheat the crab cakes and serve with the sauce and lemon wedges (if using).

- **Storage:** Store in the refrigerator for up to 5 days or in the freezer for up to 3 months. Thaw in the refrigerator overnight. To reheat, bake in an oven or toaster oven at 325°F for about 10 minutes.

- **Cooking tip:** If you can, consider forming the crab cakes the day before you cook them. It will help blend the flavors nicely and improve their structure.

  Per Serving: Calories: 319; Total fat: 10g; Carbohydrates: 30g; Fiber: 3.5g; Protein: 28g; Calcium: 251mg; Vitamin D: 10 IU; Potassium: 428mg; Magnesium: 33mg; Sodium: 691mg

BETTER-FOR-YOU FISH AND CHIPS

Serves 5

Prep time: 20 minutes • **Cook time:** 20 to 30 minutes

NUT-FREE OPTION (SEE TIP)

Comfort food doesn't need to be filled with saturated fat and salt. This DASH-friendly spin on the classic, fish and chips, ditches the traditional deep-fried aspect but retains all the flavor. Cod maintains its dense, flaky flesh when roasted in the oven. Adding a few fresh herbs, bread crumbs, and almonds enhances the fish's mild flavor. This recipe also works well in an air fryer, if you have one, adding a little extra crisp (see cooking tip on page 160).

---

2 large sweet potatoes, cut crosswise into
⅟₄-inch-thick rounds

2 tablespoons extra-virgin olive oil, divided

1 tablespoon fresh rosemary leaves

½ teaspoon salt

¼ teaspoon freshly ground black pepper

¼ cup whole wheat flour

1 large egg

2 tablespoons 1% milk

½ cup dried unseasoned bread crumbs

¼ cup slivered almonds

¼ teaspoon lemon pepper

1 teaspoon chopped fresh parsley, plus more
for serving

5 (4-ounce) fresh or (thawed) frozen cod fillets

Lemon wedges (optional)

1. Position racks in the upper and lower thirds of the oven and preheat the oven to 450°F. Line 2 sheet pans with aluminum foil.

2. In a medium bowl, toss the sweet potatoes with 1 tablespoon of oil and the rosemary. Season with the salt and pepper. Arrange in an even layer on one prepared sheet pan. Bake on the top rack, turning once, for 20 to 30 minutes, or until browned.

3. Set up a dredging station: Put the flour in a small bowl. In a second small bowl, whisk together the egg and milk. In a third, combine the bread crumbs, almonds, lemon pepper, and parsley. Coat each cod fillet in the flour, then the egg wash, then the bread crumb mixture. Arrange on the second prepared sheet pan and drizzle with the remaining 1 tablespoon of oil.

4. Bake the cod on the bottom rack for about 15 minutes, or until crisp and just cooked through.

5. Portion the cod and sweet potatoes into 5 divided storage containers; fish on one side, chips on the other.

6. To serve, after reheating the dish, top with parsley. Serve with lemon wedges (if using).

Continued ❯

- **Storage:** Store in the refrigerator for up to 1 week or in the freezer for up to 3 months. To reheat from the refrigerator, put the fish and chips on a sheet pan and bake in a 375°F oven for 8 to 12 minutes. To reheat from the freezer, thaw in the refrigerator overnight, then follow the refrigerated instructions.

- **Cooking tip:** To make these in an air fryer, set the temperature to 400°F and preheat. Working in batches, cook the sweet potatoes in a single layer for 5 to 10 minutes, or until tender. Toss to redistribute, then cook for an additional 5 to 10 minutes, or until lightly browned and crisp. Remove and cover with aluminum foil to keep warm. Place the cod in the basket, making sure the pieces are not touching one another, and fry. After 5 minutes, flip each piece of cod and continue cooking for an additional 5 minutes.

- **Nut-free option:** Substitute almonds with sunflower seeds.

  Per Serving: Calories: 301; Total fat: 10g; Carbohydrates: 27g; Fiber: 4g; Protein: 24g; Calcium: 94mg; Vitamin D: 47 IU; Potassium: 503mg; Magnesium: 76mg; Sodium: 411mg

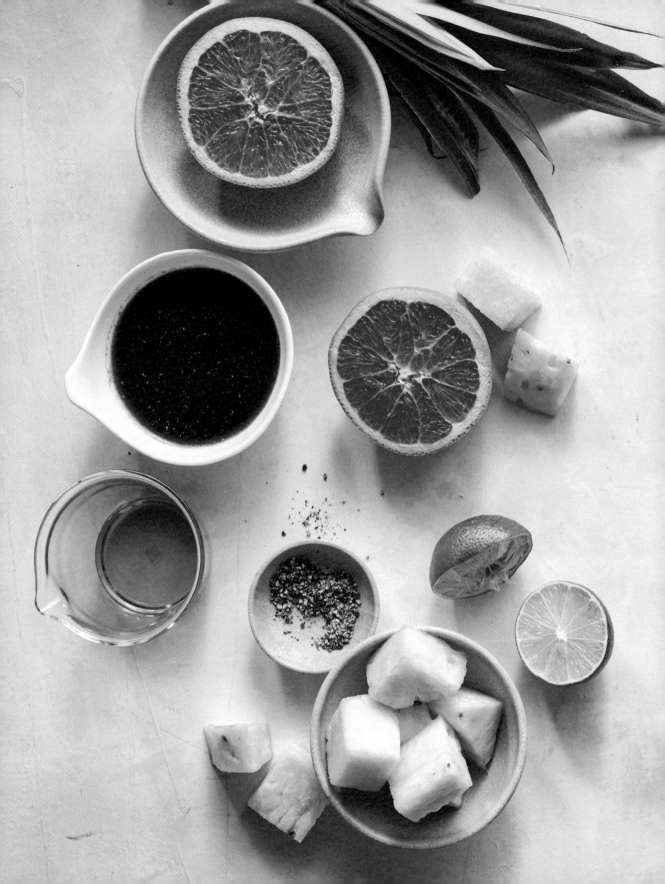

Grapefruit and
Herb Chicken
Page 164

CHAPTER 8

Poultry & Meat Mains

GRAPEFRUIT AND HERB CHICKEN

Serves 4
Prep time: 10 minutes • **Cook time:** 40 minutes
DAIRY-FREE • EGG-FREE • GLUTEN-FREE • NUT-FREE

If you find yourself getting bored with your usual chicken dishes, this flavorful combination of grapefruit and herbs is a great addition to your meal rotation. When salt is not the main seasoning for your meal, the right combination of herbs and flavorings—in this case citrus, basil, rosemary, thyme, and parsley—elevates this dish from ordinary to mouthwatering.

Nonstick cooking spray
¼ cup extra-virgin olive oil
2 tablespoons honey
2 garlic cloves, minced
Zest and juice of 1 large lemon
Zest and juice of ½ medium grapefruit
½ teaspoon dried basil

½ teaspoon dried rosemary
¼ teaspoon dried thyme
2 tablespoons chopped fresh parsley
4 (4-ounce) chicken breast cutlets, thinly sliced
¼ teaspoon salt
½ teaspoon freshly ground black pepper

1. Preheat the oven to 425°F. Coat a 9-by-13-inch baking dish with cooking spray.
2. In a large resealable bag, mix together the oil, honey, garlic, lemon zest, lemon juice, grapefruit zest, grapefruit juice, basil, rosemary, thyme, and parsley. Seal and shake until well combined.
3. Put the chicken cutlets in the bag. Seal and shake until the chicken is well coated with the marinade.
4. Transfer the chicken and the marinade to the prepared baking dish. Sprinkle the chicken with the salt and pepper. Bake for 30 to 40 minutes, or until the chicken is no longer pink in the middle. Let cool, then divide among 4 storage containers (including the juices from the baking dish).

- **Storage:** Store in the refrigerator for up to 5 days or in the freezer for up to 3 months. To reheat, vent the lid slightly, and microwave on medium for 2 minutes. From frozen, microwave on medium for 4 minutes.

- **Cooking tip:** If you have time, let the chicken breast marinate in the refrigerator from 30 minutes to 4 hours to enhance the flavor.

  Per Serving: Calories: 278; Total fat: 16g; Carbohydrates: 10g; Fiber: 0.5g; Protein: 23g; Calcium: 23mg; Vitamin D: 4 IU; Potassium: 218mg; Magnesium: 24mg; Sodium: 202mg

BAKED RANCH CHICKEN THIGHS

Serves 8
Prep time: 10 minutes • **Cook time:** 35 minutes
EGG-FREE • NUT-FREE

Chicken thighs are a moist, flavorful, and budget-friendly meat. They are a nice alternative to the breast, offering a little more fat, but not too much. The buttermilk powder here offers a bit of tang, the bread crumbs make the chicken nice and crunchy, and the seasoning mix gives it a kick. These delicious thighs pair nicely with Mashed Sweet Potatoes (page 111) or Kale-Poppy Seed Salad (page 119).

Nonstick cooking spray (optional)
2 tablespoons dried parsley
2 teaspoons dried dill
2 teaspoons dried basil
2 teaspoons garlic powder
2 teaspoons onion powder

1 teaspoon freshly ground black pepper
1 teaspoon dried chives
¼ cup dried buttermilk powder
½ cup dried unseasoned bread crumbs
8 (4-ounce) boneless, skinless chicken thighs
1 tablespoon extra-virgin olive oil

1. Preheat the oven to 400°F. Line a sheet pan with aluminum foil or coat with nonstick cooking spray.
2. In a small bowl, mix together the parsley, dill, basil, garlic powder, onion powder, pepper, chives, buttermilk powder, and bread crumbs.
3. Pat the chicken thighs dry with a paper towel. Lightly coat both sides of the chicken thighs with the oil. Dip the chicken in the seasoned bread crumbs to coat both sides. Arrange on the prepared sheet pan.
4. Cook for about 35 minutes, or until the internal temperature of the chicken has reached 165°F. Let cool, then divide among 8 storage containers.

- **Storage:** Store in the refrigerator for up to 5 days or in the freezer for up to 3 months. To reheat, microwave for 1 to 2 minutes or bake at 325°F for up to 15 minutes. To reheat from the freezer, microwave on medium for 3 to 4 minutes, or thaw in the refrigerator overnight and bake per instructions for refrigerated.

Per Serving: Calories: 202; Total fat: 8.5g; Carbohydrates: 8g; Fiber: 0.5g; Protein: 22g; Calcium: 69mg; Vitamin D: 6 IU; Potassium: 293mg; Magnesium: 26mg; Sodium: 142mg

BREADED AND BAKED CHICKEN TENDERS

Serves 4
Prep time: 10 minutes • **Cook time:** 20 minutes
NUT-FREE

This is a DASH spin on a classic that is beloved by kids and adults alike. Best of all, it's fast and pairs well with almost anything. Try it with the Mashed Sweet Potatoes (page 111) or for a new take on chicken and waffles, pair them with the Blueberry Waffles (page 88). These also cook well in an air fryer (see cooking tip).

Nonstick cooking spray
¼ cup whole wheat flour
¼ teaspoon salt
2 large eggs
1 cup dried unseasoned bread crumbs

¼ cup grated Parmesan cheese
¼ teaspoon paprika
¼ teaspoon garlic powder
1 pound chicken tenders

1. Preheat the oven to 400°F. Line a large sheet pan with foil and coat with nonstick cooking spray.
2. Set up a dredging station: In a shallow dish, mix together the flour and salt. In a small bowl, beat the eggs. In a second shallow dish, mix the bread crumbs, Parmesan, paprika, and garlic.
3. Dip each tender in the flour mixture, then the egg wash, then the bread crumb mixture until covered on both sides. Try to use one hand for dry dipping, and one for dipping in the egg to prevent a gummy mess. Arrange the tenders on the prepared sheet pan.
4. Bake for 15 to 20 minutes, or until the coating is golden brown and the chicken is no longer pink in the center, turning once halfway through. Divide among 4 storage containers.

- **Storage:** Store in the refrigerator for up to 5 days or in the freezer for up to 3 months. To reheat, bake in the oven or a toaster oven at 350°F for 3 to 4 minutes. To reheat from the freezer, microwave for 2 minutes and bake in the oven at 350°F for an additional 2 to 3 minutes.

- **Cooking tip:** To make these in an air fryer, set the temperature to 400°F and preheat. Place the chicken in the basket. Make sure the chicken pieces are not touching one another. After 5 minutes, flip each piece of chicken and continue cooking for an additional 5 minutes.

Per Serving: Calories: 328; Total fat: 14g; Carbohydrates: 21g; Fiber: 1.5g; Protein: 31g; Calcium: 103mg; Vitamin D: 22 IU; Potassium: 258mg; Magnesium: 36mg; Sodium: 419mg

STUFFED CHICKEN BREASTS WITH GARLIC MUSHROOMS AND ZESTY SPINACH

Serves 4

Prep time: 15 minutes • **Cook time:** 35 minutes

EGG-FREE • GLUTEN-FREE • NUT-FREE

Stuffed chicken breasts reinvent your dinner routine by allowing you to cook everything together. The flavors from the vegetable sauté also soak into the chicken as it bakes. Here, we build the flavor with aromatic garlic, earthy mushrooms, and bright citrus zest. This dish makes for a pretty presentation, whether serving guests or just yourself. For an easy weeknight dinner, pair with brown or wild rice.

Nonstick cooking spray (optional)

2 (8-ounce) boneless, skinless chicken breasts

3 tablespoons extra-virgin olive oil, divided

2 garlic cloves, chopped

12 small cremini mushrooms, sliced

2 cups baby spinach, chopped

¼ teaspoon freshly ground black pepper

¼ cup grated Parmesan cheese

Zest of 1 large lemon, divided

3 teaspoons fresh lemon juice, divided

1. Preheat the oven to 375°F. Line a sheet pan with aluminum foil or coat with nonstick cooking spray.
2. Working from the thickest part of each breast, cut an opening about 3 inches wide, then cut three-quarters of the way through the breast to create a pocket. Do not cut all the way through the chicken or the stuffing will spill out.
3. In a skillet, heat 2 tablespoons of oil over medium-high heat. Add the garlic and stir frequently for 30 seconds to 1 minute. Add the mushrooms and cook for about 2 minutes, or until tender. Add the spinach and stir for about 1 minute, or until wilted. Season with the pepper.
4. Transfer the cooked vegetables to a medium bowl. Add the Parmesan cheese, half of the lemon zest, and 1½ teaspoons of lemon juice. Divide the filling into 2 portions and stuff each chicken breast.

Continued ❯

STUFFED CHICKEN BREASTS WITH GARLIC MUSHROOMS
AND ZESTY SPINACH   *Continued*

5. In a small bowl, stir together the remaining 1 tablespoon of oil and the remaining 1½ teaspoons of lemon juice. Brush on top of each chicken breast.

6. Bake for about 35 minutes, or until the internal temperature of the chicken reaches 165°F. Let cool, top with remaining lemon zest, then cut each stuffed breast in half and divide into 4 storage containers.

- **Storage:** Store in the refrigerator for up to 5 days or in the freezer for up to 3 months. To reheat, microwave for 1 to 2 minutes, or bake at 325°F for up to 15 minutes. To reheat from frozen, microwave on medium for about 4 minutes.

- **Cooking tip:** Topping the chicken with oil keeps it from drying out. It also helps the chicken brown, giving it delicious color and flavor.

Per Serving: Calories: 254; Total fat: 14g; Carbohydrates: 5g; Fiber: 1g; Protein: 27g; Calcium: 94mg; Vitamin D: 6 IU; Potassium: 473mg; Magnesium: 49mg; Sodium: 170mg

CHEESY BROCCOLI AND CHICKEN BAKE

Serves 6

Prep time: 15 minutes • **Cook time:** 25 minutes

EGG-FREE • GLUTEN-FREE • NUT-FREE

This is a great recipe to have on hand when you have company or extra guests over for dinner. (Kids love it, too.) The combination of protein, whole grains, and vegetables makes this easy-to-bake meal a great addition to your weeknight rotation.

Nonstick cooking spray

2 tablespoons extra-virgin olive oil

1 pound boneless, skinless chicken breasts, cubed

4 garlic cloves, minced

1 small onion, thinly sliced

¼ teaspoon freshly ground black pepper

2 cups brown rice

4½ cups unsalted chicken stock

1½ large heads broccoli, cut into bite-size florets

1 cup nonfat plain Greek yogurt

1½ teaspoons Dijon mustard

1½ cups reduced-fat shredded Cheddar cheese

1. Preheat the oven to 400°F. Coat a 9-by-13-inch baking dish with cooking spray.
2. In a large skillet, heat the oil over medium heat. Add the chicken, garlic, onion, and pepper. Sauté while stirring for about 5 minutes. Add the rice and chicken stock and stir. Increase the heat to high and bring to a boil.
3. Pour the chicken and rice mixture into the prepared baking dish. Arrange the broccoli on top and spread evenly. Do not mix in. Cover with a lid or aluminum foil. Bake for 40 to 45 minutes.
4. Meanwhile, in a small bowl, blend together the yogurt and mustard.
5. Remove the baking dish from the oven. Uncover and stir in the yogurt and mustard mixture. Sprinkle the Cheddar cheese on top. Return to the oven and bake uncovered for 5 to 10 minutes, or until the cheese has melted. Let cool, then divide among 6 storage containers.

- **Storage:** Store in the refrigerator for up to 5 days or in the freezer up to 3 months. To reheat, vent the lid slightly, and microwave on medium for 2 minutes. To reheat from the freezer, thaw in the refrigerator overnight, or bake at 375°F for 10 minutes.

- **Substitution tip:** If you don't have broccoli, frozen green beans are a great swap.

Per Serving: Calories: 531; Total fat: 19g; Carbohydrates: 52g; Fiber: 3.5g; Protein: 39g; Calcium: 341mg; Vitamin D: 4 IU; Potassium: 600mg; Magnesium: 115mg; Sodium: 347mg

BARBECUE TURKEY BREAST

Serves 8
Prep time: 5 minutes • **Cook time:** 1 hour to 1 hour 15 minutes
DAIRY-FREE • EGG-FREE • GLUTEN-FREE • NUT-FREE

Barbecue seasoning brings a lot of flavor but leaves behind salt, making it perfect for DASH. Pairing new spice blends with family-favorite meats like turkey breast is a great way to embrace something new. This recipe also goes well with our jerk seasoning (see page 154) or ranch seasoning (see page 165).

Nonstick cooking spray (optional)

¼ cup packed brown sugar

2 teaspoons garlic powder

2 teaspoons onion powder

1 teaspoon paprika

1 teaspoon freshly ground black pepper

1 teaspoon mustard powder

½ teaspoon chili powder (optional)

¼ teaspoon cayenne pepper

3 pounds boneless turkey breast

1. Preheat the oven to 350°F. Line a roasting pan with aluminum foil or coat with nonstick cooking spray.
2. In a small bowl, mix together the brown sugar, garlic powder, onion powder, paprika, black pepper, mustard powder, chili powder (if using), and cayenne pepper. Season the turkey breast with this rub and transfer to the prepared roasting pan.
3. Cover the turkey with foil to avoid browning. Roast for 40 minutes. Then begin checking the turkey breast every 10 to 15 minutes until the internal temperature of the turkey breast has reached 165°F. Let rest for 5 minutes before slicing. Portion the turkey into 8 storage containers.

- **Storage:** Store in the refrigerator for up to 4 days or in the freezer for up to 2 months. To reheat, microwave for 1 to 2 minutes, or bake at 325°F for 15 minutes. To reheat from the freezer, microwave for 3 to 4 minutes.

- **Ingredient tip:** This rub tastes great on a whole turkey as well. When cooking a turkey, allow 20 minutes per pound, and baste every 15 to 20 minutes. Consider cooking the turkey upside down for the first 30 minutes to add juiciness to the white meat.

Per Serving: Calories: 233; Total fat: 3g; Carbohydrates: 8g; Fiber: 0.5g; Protein: 41g; Calcium: 21mg; Vitamin D: 13 IU; Potassium: 365mg; Magnesium: 45mg; Sodium: 136mg

TURKEY CHILI

Serves 6

Prep time: 10 minutes • **Cook time:** 45 minutes

DAIRY-FREE • EGG-FREE • GLUTEN-FREE • NUT-FREE

This delicious, one-pot meal is simple, unfussy, and a DASH-friendly comfort food. High in protein and rich in fiber, it is one of Maria-Paula's go-to fall meals—though it's great all year round.

1½ teaspoons extra-virgin olive oil

1 medium onion, chopped

1 red bell pepper, chopped

3 garlic cloves, minced

1 pound extra-lean ground turkey

1½ cups unsalted chicken stock

1 (15-ounce) can no-salt-added kidney beans, drained and rinsed

1 (15-ounce) can no-salt-added corn kernels

1 (28-ounce) can no-salt-added diced tomatoes

2 teaspoons chili powder

1½ teaspoons ground cumin

1 teaspoon dried oregano

½ teaspoon paprika

½ teaspoon salt

½ teaspoon freshly ground black pepper

¼ teaspoon cayenne pepper

Unsalted corn chips, shredded reduced-fat cheese or reduced-fat sour cream, and cubed avocado, for topping (optional)

1. In a large pot, heat the oil over medium heat. Add the onion, bell pepper, and garlic and sauté, stirring regularly, for about 5 minutes, or until softened.
2. Add the turkey and cook, making sure to break up the meat, until it evenly browns. Pour in the chicken stock, beans, corn, and tomatoes. Stir well.
3. Stir in the chili powder, cumin, oregano, paprika, salt, black pepper, and cayenne pepper. Bring to a boil, then reduce the heat to a simmer, cover, and cook for 30 minutes to blend the flavors. Let cool, then divide into 6 storage containers. Top with chips, cheese, and avocado (if using).

- **Storage:** Store in the refrigerator for up to 5 days or in the freezer for up to 3 months. To reheat from the refrigerator, vent the lid slightly, and microwave on medium for 2 minutes. To reheat from the freezer, microwave on medium for 3 minutes, stir, and microwave an additional 1 to 2 minutes.

  Per Serving (without toppings): Calories: 257; Total fat: 3g; Carbohydrates: 32g; Fiber: 9.5g; Protein: 27g; Calcium: 97mg; Vitamin D: 11 IU; Potassium: 939mg; Magnesium: 62mg; Sodium: 286mg

PULLED PORK

Serves 4
Prep time: 5 minutes • **Cook time:** 8 hours
DAIRY-FREE • EGG-FREE • GLUTEN-FREE • NUT-FREE

As Texans, we couldn't pass up an opportunity to share our favorite Southern recipe with you. A true crowd-pleaser, this pulled pork will become your go-to for days when you're short on time and energy. Use the pork in sandwiches, on top of a baked potato, or pair with the Roasted Carrots and Beets (page 105), Kale-Poppy Seed Salad (page 119), or Mashed Sweet Potatoes (page 111). Whichever way you choose, you won't be disappointed.

1 small onion, diced

2 garlic cloves, minced

1 cup unsalted chicken stock

Juice of ½ orange

1 tablespoon paprika

1 teaspoon dried oregano

1 teaspoon freshly ground black pepper

½ teaspoon ground cumin

½ teaspoon salt

2 pounds boneless pork shoulder or pork butt

1. In a slow cooker, combine the onion, garlic, chicken stock, and orange juice.
2. In a small bowl, mix together the paprika, oregano, pepper, cumin, and salt.
3. Trim any excess fat from the pork and rub the spice mix all over until it is well coated. Place it in the slow cooker on top of the onion and liquids.
4. Cover and cook on low for 8 hours, or until the meat can be pulled apart in shreds with a fork.
5. Remove the pork to a cutting board and use 2 forks to shred it. Portion the pork into 4 storage containers. Add some of the cooking liquids to each container to add moisture to the pork (good for both reheating and serving).

- **Storage:** Store in the refrigerator for up to 5 days or in the freezer for up to 3 months. To reheat, microwave on medium for 2 minutes. To reheat from the freezer, microwave on medium for 4 minutes with a splash of chicken stock.

- **Variations:** You can add reduced-sodium barbecue sauce to turn this into barbecue pulled pork.

Per Serving: Calories: 394; Total fat: 25g; Carbohydrates: 2g; Fiber: 0.5g; Protein: 37g; Calcium: 49mg; Vitamin D: 66 IU; Potassium: 462mg; Magnesium: 35mg; Sodium: 391mg

SAVORY PORK LOIN

Serves 6
Prep time: 5 minutes • **Cook time:** 25 to 30 minutes
DAIRY-FREE • EGG-FREE • GLUTEN-FREE • NUT-FREE

When eaten in moderation, pork is an excellent protein choice for the DASH diet. It's a good source of potassium, riboflavin, and zinc, as well as vitamin B_6, thiamin, phosphorus, and niacin. The loin is a great lean cut. When it comes to protein, remember that portion size is important—a serving should be about the size of your palm.

Nonstick cooking spray (optional)
1½ tablespoons fresh rosemary, chopped
1½ tablespoons fresh thyme, chopped

2 garlic cloves, minced
¼ teaspoon freshly ground black pepper
2 pounds boneless pork loin

1. Preheat the oven to 350°F. Line a roasting pan with aluminum foil or coat with nonstick cooking spray.
2. In a small bowl, mix together the rosemary, thyme, garlic, and pepper. Season the pork loin with this rub.
3. Transfer to the prepared roasting pan and bake for 25 to 30 minutes, or until the internal temperature of the pork loin has reached 145°F. Let rest for 5 minutes before slicing. Portion the pork into 6 storage containers.

- **Storage:** Store in the refrigerator for up to 4 days or in the freezer for up to 3 months. To reheat, microwave for 1 to 2 minutes, or bake at 325°F for up to 15 minutes. To reheat from the freezer, microwave on medium for 4 minutes with a splash of chicken stock.

- **Variations:** With a mild flavor, pork is a great meat to season. Consider trading this savory seasoning for the jerk seasoning from Jerk Salmon (page 154) or the barbecue seasoning from Barbecue Turkey Breast (page 170).

Per Serving: Calories: 216; Total fat: 11g; Carbohydrates: 0g; Fiber: 0g; Protein: 29g; Calcium: 15mg; Vitamin D: 24 IU; Potassium: 477mg; Magnesium: 25mg; Sodium: 72mg

HONEY-GARLIC PORK CHOPS

Serves 4
Prep time: 5 minutes • **Cook time:** 25 minutes
EGG-FREE • NUT-FREE • GLUTEN-FREE OPTION (SEE TIP)

A touch of sweetness makes this dish one you will be thinking about hours after eating it. A delicious choice for any season, we like to pair it with Mashed Sweet Potatoes (page 111) in the fall, a Simple Green Salad (page 118) in the summer, or Cilantro Rice (page 108) in the spring. Choosing center loin chops gives you the chance to enjoy an excellent source of lean protein while providing potassium, iron, and zinc.

2½ tablespoons honey

4 garlic cloves, minced

1 tablespoon reduced-sodium soy sauce

1 tablespoon no-salt-added ketchup

½ teaspoon freshly ground black pepper

½ teaspoon dried oregano

4 (6-ounce) bone-in loin pork chops, fat trimmed

1 tablespoon extra-virgin olive oil

1 tablespoon unsalted butter

1. Preheat the oven to 400°F.
2. In a small bowl, mix together the honey, garlic, soy sauce, ketchup, pepper, and oregano.
3. Put the pork chops in a large bowl and pour the sauce over them. Mix until fully coated.
4. In a large oven-safe skillet, heat the oil over medium-high heat. Add the pork chops with sauce to the skillet. Sear for about 2 minutes per side, until they brown slightly. Remove from the heat.
5. Add ¾ teaspoon of butter to the top of each pork chop. Transfer to the oven and bake for 15 to 18 minutes, or until the pork reaches an internal temperature of 145°F. Let cool, then place a chop in each of 4 storage containers. Divide the pan sauce evenly over the portions.

• **Storage:** Store in the refrigerator for up to 5 days or in the freezer for up to 3 months. To reheat, vent the lid slightly, and microwave on medium for 1½ to 2 minutes. To reheat from the freezer, add 2 tablespoons of chicken stock, and microwave on medium for 3 minutes, turn over, and microwave an additional minute.

• **Gluten-free option:** Use a gluten-free soy sauce or substitute coconut aminos for the soy sauce.

Per Serving: Calories: 271; Total fat: 14g; Carbohydrates: 13g; Fiber: 0g; Protein: 22g; Calcium: 56mg; Vitamin D: 31 IU; Potassium: 330mg; Magnesium: 22mg; Sodium: 211mg

SHEET PAN STEAKS WITH ROASTED VEGETABLES

Serves 4

Prep time: 15 minutes • **Cook time:** 35 minutes

DAIRY-FREE • EGG-FREE • GLUTEN-FREE • NUT-FREE

Size is important here; there are quite a few vegetables included, so look for at least a 12-by-17-inch sheet pan, also known as a half-sheet pan. Alternatively, you can divide the vegetables between two smaller ones. The best thing about this recipe is that cleanup is a breeze.

Nonstick cooking spray (optional)

6 medium carrots

2 medium zucchini, cut into 2-inch sections

2 medium sweet potatoes, peeled and cut into 1-inch cubes

1 tablespoon extra-virgin olive oil

¼ teaspoon garlic salt, divided

¼ teaspoon lemon pepper, divided

4 (4-ounce) sirloin steaks

1. Preheat the oven to 350°F. Line a 12-by-17-inch sheet pan with aluminum foil or coat with nonstick cooking spray.
2. Peel the carrots and cut into 2-inch sections where thin and 1-inch sections where thick. In a large bowl, toss together the carrots, zucchini, and sweet potatoes with the oil, ⅛ teaspoon of garlic salt, and ⅛ teaspoon of lemon pepper.
3. Spread the vegetables onto the prepared sheet pan and bake for 35 minutes, turning once.
4. Season both sides of the steaks with the remaining ⅛ teaspoon of garlic salt and ⅛ teaspoon of lemon pepper.
5. Add the steaks to the sheet pan. Turn the oven to broil and broil the steaks for 4 minutes per side, or until the internal temperature reaches 145°F for medium-rare.
6. Place a steak in each of 4 storage containers. Divide the vegetables into 4 separate storage containers.

- **Storage:** Store in the refrigerator for up to 5 days or in the freezer for up to 3 months. To reheat the vegetables, microwave for 30 seconds to 1 minute, or bake at 325°F for 10 minutes. To reheat the steak, bake at 325°F for 15 minutes, turning once. Or add unsalted beef stock, and microwave for 30 seconds on each side until warm, or sauté in a skillet until warm. To reheat from the freezer, add beef stock, and microwave for 1 minute on each side until warm.

Per Serving: Calories: 311; Total fat: 12g; Carbohydrates: 24g; Fiber: 5g; Protein: 27g; Calcium: 78mg; Vitamin D: 6 IU; Potassium: 975mg; Magnesium: 59mg; Sodium: 277mg

GREEK-STYLE TOP ROUND STEAKS

Serves 4
Prep time: 5 minutes • **Cook time:** 12 to 15 minutes
EGG-FREE • GLUTEN-FREE • NUT-FREE

You don't need to give up red meat on the DASH diet; it's a complete high-quality protein, one that includes all nine essential amino acids. It also features a wide variety of minerals, such as iron and selenium, and a host of B vitamins, including B_6, B_{12}, niacin, and riboflavin. What matters is how much you eat—6 ounces of lean protein per day, and beef can be part of that total. It also matters which cut you choose—leaner is better. With beef, look for sirloin or top round steak (which is what we use here); and for ground beef, look for 95 percent lean. No grill? No problem. See the cooking tip on page 177 for making this on the stovetop.

1½ teaspoons garlic powder

1½ teaspoons dried basil

1½ teaspoons dried oregano

⅛ teaspoon salt

⅛ teaspoon freshly ground black pepper

4 (4-ounce) top round steaks

Nonstick cooking spray

Zest of ½ large lemon

1 tablespoon fresh lemon juice

2 tablespoons crumbled feta cheese

1. In a small bowl, mix together the garlic powder, basil, oregano, salt, and pepper. Season the steaks on both sides.
2. Coat the grill grates with cooking spray. Preheat the grill to medium-high heat (350°F to 400°F).
3. Grill the steaks for 6 minutes on each side, or until the internal temperature reaches 135°F for medium-rare. Add a few more minutes for medium.
4. Let the steaks cool, then store them in 4 storage containers. Store the lemon zest, lemon juice, and feta cheese separately.
5. To serve, after reheating the steaks, sprinkle with lemon zest and lemon juice and top with the cheese.

- **Storage:** Store in the refrigerator for up to 4 days or in the freezer for up to 3 months. To reheat the steaks, bake at 325°F for up to 15 minutes, turning once; alternatively, add unsalted beef stock and microwave for 30 seconds on each side until warm, or sauté in a skillet until warm. To reheat from the freezer, thaw in the refrigerator overnight, and follow the refrigerated instructions.

- **Cooking tip:** To cook indoors, heat 2 teaspoons of extra-virgin olive oil in a cast-iron or non-stick skillet over high heat. Sear the steaks for 3 minutes on each side to reach an internal temperature of 135°F for medium-rare.

Per Serving: Calories: 214; Total fat: 12g; Carbohydrates: 1g; Fiber: 0.5g; Protein: 27g; Calcium: 33mg; Vitamin D: 2 IU; Potassium: 382mg; Magnesium: 16mg; Sodium: 225mg

BEEF TENDERLOIN MEDALLIONS WITH HORSERADISH YOGURT SAUCE

Serves 4
Prep time: 10 minutes • **Cook time:** 5 minutes
EGG-FREE • GLUTEN-FREE • NUT-FREE • DAIRY-FREE OPTION (SEE TIP)

How much flavor can your taste buds handle? This amazing recipe will satisfy all your senses. Full-fat yogurt adds the perfect amount of creaminess to mix nicely with the horseradish sauce, adding an extra kick of flavor to an already flavorful cut. Try this recipe with Zesty Lemon Brussels Sprouts (page 106) or a Wedge Salad with Creamy Blue Cheese Dressing (page 120).

FOR THE HORSERADISH SAUCE

¾ cup whole-milk Greek yogurt

2 tablespoons prepared horseradish

1 garlic clove, minced

¼ teaspoon freshly ground black pepper

2 teaspoons 1% milk

FOR THE MEDALLIONS

12 ounces beef tenderloin, flattened and cut into 4 pieces

½ teaspoon freshly ground black pepper

½ teaspoon garlic powder

1 tablespoon unsalted butter

TO MAKE THE HORSERADISH SAUCE

1. In a small bowl, whisk together the yogurt, horseradish, garlic, pepper, and milk until well mixed. Divide the sauce among 4 condiment cups.

TO MAKE THE MEDALLIONS

2. Season the tenderloin with the pepper and garlic powder.
3. In a large skillet, melt the butter over medium-high heat. Add the beef and sauté for about 2 minutes on each side, or until the outside is browned and the inside is very pink, medium-rare. Remove from the heat. When cool, portion the beef into 4 storage containers.
4. To serve, reheat the beef and top with horseradish sauce.

- **Storage:** Store in the refrigerator for up to 5 days or in the freezer for up to 3 months. To reheat the steak, bake at 325°F for up to 15 minutes, turning once; alternatively, add unsalted beef stock and microwave for 30 seconds on each side until warm, or sauté in a skillet until warm. To reheat from the freezer, thaw in the refrigerator overnight, and follow the refrigerated instructions.

- **Dairy-free option:** Use plain soy yogurt instead of Greek yogurt, extra-virgin olive oil instead of butter, and soy milk instead of cow's milk.

Per Serving: Calories: 185; Total fat: 9g; Carbohydrates: 3g; Fiber: 0.5g; Protein: 23g; Calcium: 72mg; Vitamin D: 3 IU; Potassium: 332mg; Magnesium: 18mg; Sodium: 87mg

Fresh Berries and Homemade Whipped Cream
Page 188

CHAPTER 9

DASH Staples, Sauces & Sweets

SWEET BALSAMIC REDUCTION

Makes about ½ cup
Prep time: 1 minute, plus 1 hour to chill • **Cook time:** 30 to 40 minutes
DAIRY-FREE • EGG-FREE • GLUTEN-FREE • NUT-FREE • VEGETARIAN

A sweet balsamic reduction is a great addition to all manner of dishes, from savory to sweet. Try it on salads—like the Apple Caprese Salad (page 58)—or use it to add just a hint of sweetness to meaty dishes like Savory Pork Loin (page 173). It's also a welcome extra to the Fresh Berries and Homemade Whipped Cream (page 188) or even just over fresh peaches with vanilla ice cream.

1 cup balsamic vinegar   2 tablespoons honey

1. In a small pot, combine the vinegar and honey. Bring to a boil. Reduce the heat to medium and simmer for 30 to 40 minutes, or until reduced by half and thickened.
2. Transfer to a jar or storage container. If not storing for future use, chill for at least 1 hour before serving.

- **Storage:** Store in the refrigerator for up to 1 month.

  Per Serving (1 tablespoon): Calories: 44; Total fat: 0g; Carbohydrates: 10g; Fiber: 0g; Protein: 0g; Calcium: 9mg; Vitamin D: 0 IU; Potassium: 39mg; Magnesium: 4mg; Sodium: 8mg

LEMON VINAIGRETTE

Makes about ¾ cup
Prep time: 5 minutes
DAIRY-FREE • EGG-FREE • GLUTEN-FREE • NUT-FREE • VEGAN

This dressing is a staple every household should have on hand. It's delicious, simple, and a great complement to a variety of salads, fish, and chicken entrées. Homemade dressings let you control the sodium, fat, and sugar.

½ cup extra-virgin olive oil

Zest of 1 large lemon

Juice of 2 large lemons

½ teaspoon Dijon mustard

2 garlic cloves, minced

¼ teaspoon freshly ground black pepper

In a small screw-top jar, combine the oil, lemon zest, lemon juice, mustard, garlic, and pepper and shake until well combined.

- **Storage:** Store in the refrigerator for up to 7 days. Always shake before serving.

- **Variations:** Many different citrus fruits make a great vinaigrette. Consider swapping out the lemon juice for grapefruit juice, orange juice, or lime juice.

  Per Serving (1 tablespoon): Calories: 83; Total fat: 9g; Carbohydrates: 1g; Fiber: 0g; Protein: 0g; Calcium: 2mg; Vitamin D: 0 IU; Potassium: 11mg; Magnesium: 1mg; Sodium: 5mg

GREEK YOGURT DILL DRESSING

Makes 1 cup
Prep time: 5 minutes
EGG-FREE • GLUTEN-FREE • NUT-FREE • VEGETARIAN

This creamy dressing can be used in a variety of ways. The Greek yogurt provides a nice texture while the dill gives it a comforting flavor. In addition to salads, use this to add moisture or flavor to meats. It can also be used as a vegetable dip or a spread for sandwiches.

---

2 tablespoons minced fresh chives
2 tablespoons fresh lime juice
¾ cup nonfat plain Greek yogurt

2 tablespoons chopped fresh dill
1 garlic clove, minced

In a small bowl, combine the chives and lime juice and let sit for 5 minutes. Mix in the yogurt, dill, and garlic.

- **Storage:** Store in a mason jar in the refrigerator for up to 5 days.

- **Substitution tip:** Swap in 2 tablespoons each of freeze-dried chives and dill for the fresh herbs.

    Per Serving (2 tablespoons): Calories: 15; Total fat: 0g; Carbohydrates: 1.5g; Fiber: 0g; Protein: 2g; Calcium: 27mg; Vitamin D: 0 IU; Potassium: 42mg; Magnesium: 3mg; Sodium: 8mg

GREEN GODDESS DRESSING

Makes about 1½ cups
Prep time: 15 minutes, plus 1 hour to chill
EGG-FREE • GLUTEN-FREE • NUT-FREE • VEGETARIAN

Named for its signature hue, green goddess dressing first appeared at the Palace Hotel in San Francisco in 1923. Originally a combination of anchovies, mayonnaise, scallions, parsley, tarragon, vinegar, and chives, the dressing has evolved and now encompasses a variety of different ingredients in different recipes; some even call for avocado. Here, we add protein with Greek yogurt. The tint remains the same.

1 cup nonfat plain Greek yogurt
Juice of 1 large lemon
2 tablespoons fresh tarragon leaves

2 tablespoons chopped fresh basil
1 scallion, chopped
¼ teaspoon freshly ground black pepper

1. In a blender, combine the yogurt, lemon juice, tarragon, basil, scallion, and pepper and blend until smooth.
2. Transfer to a jar or storage container and refrigerate for at least 1 hour before serving.

- **Storage:** Store in the refrigerator for up to 5 days.

- **Variations:** Make this dressing a little more savory and earthy by changing out the lemon and basil for minced garlic, fresh parsley, and Parmesan cheese.

Per Serving (2 tablespoons): Calories: 14; Total fat: 0g; Carbohydrates: 1g; Fiber: 0g; Protein: 2g; Calcium: 26mg; Vitamin D: 0 IU; Potassium: 45mg; Magnesium: 4mg; Sodium: 8mg

BLACK BEAN HUMMUS

Serves 8
Prep time: 5 minutes • **Cook time:** 5 minutes
DAIRY-FREE • EGG-FREE • GLUTEN-FREE • NUT-FREE • VEGAN

Everyone will want more of this delicious yet nutritious dip. Swapping out traditional chick-peas for black beans allows a twist on flavors and an increase in antioxidants. Add a little variety to your appetizers with this crowd-pleasing dip served with toasted pita bread and fresh veggies. Or use it as a spread on a vegetable sandwich.

⅓ cup fresh cilantro leaves
1 garlic clove, peeled
1 (15-ounce) can no-salt-added black beans, drained and rinsed
6 Kalamata olives, pitted
2 tablespoons fresh lime juice

2 tablespoons tahini
1 tablespoon extra-virgin olive oil
¾ teaspoon ground cumin
¼ teaspoon paprika
¼ teaspoon salt

In a food processor, combine the cilantro, garlic, beans, olives, lime juice, tahini, oil, cumin, paprika, and salt. Transfer to a storage container.

- **Storage:** Store in the refrigerator for up to 7 days.

  Per Serving: Calories: 94; Total fat: 5g; Carbohydrates: 9g; Fiber: 3g; Protein: 4g; Calcium: 33mg; Vitamin D: 0 IU; Potassium: 149mg; Magnesium: 30mg; Sodium: 126mg

SIMPLE TOMATO SAUCE

Makes 2 cups
Prep time: 10 minutes • **Cook time:** 20 minutes
DAIRY-FREE • EGG-FREE • GLUTEN-FREE • NUT-FREE • VEGAN

This is a departure from your typical tomato sauce. We use grape tomatoes to create a slightly sweet, slightly acidic flavor. They are halved before cooking so they become soft and ready to mix with any pasta. You can easily swap out grape tomatoes for another variety, depending on how you'd like to change the sauce. Campari provides sweetness, yellow tomatoes provide a milder flavor, and heirlooms add flavors that match their color palette—green tomatoes have an acidic, lemon-like flavor; black or purple tomatoes bring a smoky sweetness; and orange tomatoes offer a sweeter, milder flavor.

¼ cup extra-virgin olive oil

3 garlic cloves, minced

2 pints grape tomatoes, halved

2 tablespoons chopped fresh basil

¼ teaspoon salt

¼ teaspoon freshly ground black pepper

¼ teaspoon red pepper flakes (optional)

1. In a large skillet, heat the oil over medium heat. Add the garlic and cook, stirring constantly, for 30 seconds to 1 minute. Stir in the tomatoes. Reduce the heat slightly and stir in the basil, salt, and pepper. Cook, stirring occasionally, for about 20 minutes, or until the tomatoes are softened and the sauce has thickened slightly.
2. Stir in the red pepper flakes (if using). Remove from the heat. Let cool, then portion into 4 small storage containers. Give your sauce a little room to breathe by selecting a container that will hold 6 ounces or more.

- **Storage:** Store in the refrigerator for up to 5 days or in the freezer for up to 3 months. To thaw, refrigerate overnight. Reheat on the stovetop over medium heat until warm.

- **Cooking tip:** When freezing foods in mason jars or any other glass container, do not fill to the top. This will allow for expansion. You might also want to consider freezing without the lids or placing them on loosely and tightening them the next day.

    Per Serving (½ cup): Calories: 153; Total fat: 14g; Carbohydrates: 15g; Fiber: 2g; Protein: 2g; Calcium: 6mg; Vitamin D: 0 IU; Potassium: 13mg; Magnesium: 1mg; Sodium: 176mg

FRESH BERRIES AND HOMEMADE WHIPPED CREAM

Serves 6
Prep time: 15 minutes
EGG-FREE • GLUTEN-FREE • NUT-FREE • VEGETARIAN

Homemade whipped cream is simple to make and better for you than store-bought options, since there are no processed ingredients and you control the amount of sugar added. It's also a breeze with the right equipment and technique. Using a cold bowl is key; it allows air bubbles to expand at just the right time to create a light airy mass. Pay attention to your peaks—you want them slightly soft and a little stiff. Whisk too much, and you'll make butter.

---

1 cup cold heavy cream
2 tablespoons sugar
½ teaspoon vanilla extract

1 cup blueberries
1 cup raspberries
1 cup strawberries, hulled and sliced

1. Chill a metal bowl and metal whisk in the freezer for 10 to 15 minutes. You can also use a stand mixer, but put the bowl and whisk attachment in the freezer.
2. In the chilled bowl, combine the cream, sugar, and vanilla. Whip until you see soft peaks. Whisk just a little more until the peaks are stiff. Divide the whipped cream among 6 storage containers.
3. In a large bowl, mix together the blueberries, raspberries, and strawberries. Divide evenly into 6 storage containers.
4. Serve the fruit topped with the whipped cream.

- **Storage:** Store in the refrigerator for up to 3 days. When ready to serve, whisk the cream again for 10 to 15 seconds.

- **Ingredient tip:** One of the great things about the DASH diet is that it allows for sweets throughout the week. Focus on pairing nutrient-rich fruits like berries with something a little more indulgent like whipped cream. It allows you to satisfy your sweet tooth without eating too many calories.

Per Serving: Calories: 185; Total fat: 15g; Carbohydrates: 13g; Fiber: 2.5g; Protein: 2g; Calcium: 37mg; Vitamin D: 25 IU; Potassium: 125mg; Magnesium: 12mg; Sodium: 12mg

FRESH FRUIT WITH CHOCOLATE-PEANUT BUTTER DRIZZLE

Serves 6

Prep time: 5 minutes, plus 1 hour to chill • **Cook time:** 5 minutes

EGG-FREE • GLUTEN-FREE • VEGETARIAN • DAIRY-FREE/VEGAN OPTION (SEE TIP)

The DASH diet focuses on nutrient-rich foods first, but that doesn't mean a little bit of indulgence isn't allowed from time to time. The dark chocolate helps satisfy your cravings for something sweet without going overboard, and the apple provides a nice crunch. As with all foods, it's about portion control. With these four slices per serving, you get mostly fruit and a drizzle of deliciousness.

---

2 ounces dark chocolate chips

2 tablespoons creamy peanut butter

2 medium apples, cut into 24 slices

1. In a small bowl, mix together the chocolate chips and peanut butter. Microwave on high for 30 seconds and stir. Continue to heat in 30-second intervals, stirring after each, until melted.

2. Line a sheet pan with wax paper. Arrange the apple slices on the prepared pan and drizzle the chocolate–peanut butter mixture over the slices. Chill in the refrigerator for 1 hour to firm up. Place 2 apple slices in each of 6 small storage containers.

- **Storage:** Store in the refrigerator for up to 3 days.

- **Variations:** If you don't have apples on hand, you could also drizzle the sauce over unsalted pretzel sticks.

- **Dairy-free/vegan option:** Use vegan chocolate chips.

Per Serving (4 slices): Calories: 108; Total fat: 6.5g; Carbohydrates: 15g; Fiber: 3g; Protein: 2g; Calcium: 6mg; Vitamin D: 0 IU; Potassium: 95mg; Magnesium: 12mg; Sodium: 23mg

LEMON-ZUCCHINI CAKE

Serves 12
Prep time: 15 minutes • **Cook time:** 55 minutes
NUT-FREE • VEGETARIAN • GLUTEN-FREE OPTION (SEE TIP)

You will be surprised how well a vegetable works in a cake. It's a fantastic way to add mois-ture and sweetness. Serve it with a cup of coffee for breakfast or a cup of tea for a snack. Adding Greek yogurt and applesauce make this recipe lower in fat but still very moist.

FOR THE CAKE

Nonstick cooking spray

1¼ cups all-purpose flour, plus more for dusting

1 teaspoon baking powder

½ teaspoon baking soda

¼ teaspoon salt

4 tablespoons (½ stick) unsalted butter, at
    room temperature

1½ cups unsweetened applesauce

1 cup sugar

2 tablespoons honey

½ teaspoon vanilla extract

3 large eggs

5 ounces nonfat plain Greek yogurt

Zest of 2 large lemons

¼ cup fresh lemon juice

1 large zucchini, shredded

FOR THE GLAZE (OPTIONAL)

½ cup powdered sugar

Zest and juice of 1 large lemon

TO MAKE THE CAKE

1. Preheat the oven to 350°F. Coat a Bundt pan (or a 9-by-13-inch cake pan) with cooking spray and dust with a little flour.

2. In a small bowl, mix together the flour, baking powder, baking soda, and salt. Set aside.

3. In a large bowl, with an electric mixer (or by hand), beat the butter for about 1 minute. Add the applesauce and continue beating. Little by little, add the sugar, honey, vanilla, and eggs, beating until well combined.

4. Gradually (and on low speed if using a mixer), add the flour mixture to the wet ingredients in 3 additions, alternating with the yogurt, beginning and ending with the flour. Stop beating. Fold in the lemon zest, lemon juice, and zucchini with a spoon until well combined.

5. Spoon the mixture into the prepared pan. Bake for about 50 minutes, or until a toothpick inserted into the center of the cake comes out clean. Allow it to cool completely in the pan. If not making the glaze, cut into 12 wedges (for the Bundt) or 12 squares (if in a cake pan) and store each in a storage container.

TO MAKE THE GLAZE

6. In a small bowl, mix together the powdered sugar, lemon zest, and lemon juice.
7. Invert the Bundt pan over a large plate and drizzle the cake evenly with the glaze. If in a cake pan, drizzle the glaze over the cake still in the pan. Let the glaze set.
8. Slice the cake into 12 wedges or squares and store each in a separate storage container.

- **Storage:** Store in the refrigerator for up to 5 days. Allow to sit at room temperature for 10 minutes before serving.

- **Gluten-free option:** Use all-purpose gluten-free flour.

  Per Serving (unglazed): Calories: 216; Total fat: 8g; Carbohydrates: 34g; Fiber: 1g; Protein: 5g; Calcium: 29mg; Vitamin D: 10 IU; Potassium: 144mg; Magnesium: 12mg; Sodium: 74mg

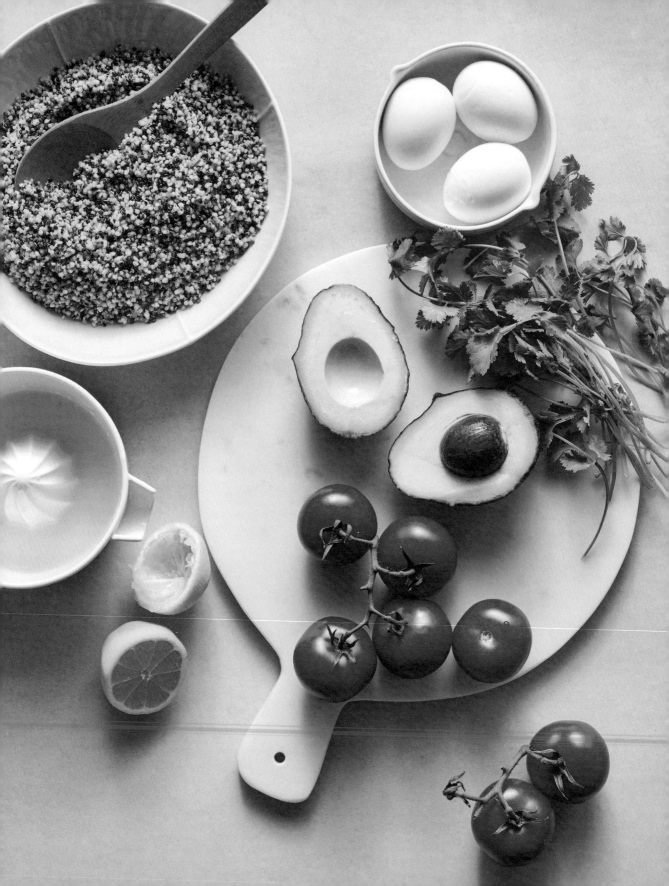

MEASUREMENT CONVERSIONS

Volume Equivalents (Liquid)

US Standard	US Standard (ounces)	Metric (approximate)
2 tablespoons	1 fl. oz.	30 mL
¼ cup	2 fl. oz.	60 mL
½ cup	4 fl. oz.	120 mL
1 cup	8 fl. oz.	240 mL
1½ cups	12 fl. oz.	355 mL
2 cups or 1 pint	16 fl. oz.	475 mL
4 cups or 1 quart	32 fl. oz.	1 L
1 gallon	128 fl. oz.	4 L

Oven Temperatures

Fahrenheit (F)	Celsius (C) (approximate)
250°F	120°C
300°F	150°C
325°F	165°C
350°F	180°C
375°F	190°C
400°F	200°C
425°F	220°C
450°F	230°C

Volume Equivalents (Dry)

US Standard	Metric (approximate)
1/8 teaspoon	0.5 mL
¼ teaspoon	1 mL
½ teaspoon	2 mL
¾ teaspoon	4 mL
1 teaspoon	5 mL
1 tablespoon	15 mL
¼ cup	59 mL
1/3 cup	79 mL
½ cup	118 mL
2/3 cup	156 mL
¾ cup	177 mL
1 cup	235 mL
2 cups or 1 pint	475 mL
3 cups	700 mL
4 cups or 1 quart	1 L

Weight Equivalents

US Standard	Metric (approximate)
½ ounce	15 g
1 ounce	30 g
2 ounces	60 g
4 ounces	115 g
8 ounces	225 g
12 ounces	340 g
16 ounces or 1 pound	455 g

REFERENCES

American Heart Association. "High Blood Pressure." Accessed January 29, 2020. Heart.org/en/health-topics/high-blood-pressure.

American Heart Association. "The Salty Six." Accessed January 29, 2020. Heart.org/en/healthy-living/healthy-eating/eat-smart/sodium/salty-six-infographic.

Appel L. et al. "A Clinical Trial of the Effects of Dietary Patterns on Blood Pressure." *New England Journal of Medicine* 336, no. 16 (April 1997): 1117–24. doi: 10.1056/NEJM199704173361601.

Campbell, A. "DASH Eating Plan: An Eating Pattern for Diabetes Management." *Diabetes Spectrum* 30, no. 2 (May 2017): 76–81. doi: 10.2337/ds16-0084.

Centers for Disease Control and Prevention. "Hypertension Statistics and Maps." Accessed April 23, 2020. CDC.gov/bloodpressure/facts.htm.

Chiu, S. et al. "Comparison of the DASH (Dietary Approaches to Stop Hypertension) diet and a higher-fat DASH diet on blood pressure and lipids and lipoproteins: a randomized controlled trial." American Journal of Clinical Nutrition, 103, no. 2 (February 2016): 341–347.

Dietary Guidelines for Americans 2015–2020, 8th edition. (Washington, DC: US Department of Health and Human Services and US Department of Agriculture, 2015). Health.gov/dietaryguidelines/2015/guidelines.

Fridge & Freezer Storage Chart. (Washington, DC: US Food and Drug Administration, 2018). FDA.gov/media/74435/download.

Hinderliter, A. et al. "The Long-Term Effects of Lifestyle Change on Blood Pressure: One-Year Follow-up of the ENCORE Study." *American Journal of Hypertension* 27, no. 5 (May 2014): 734–41. doi: 10.1093/ajh/hpt183.

Lin, P. et al. "The DASH Diet and Sodium Reduction Improve Markers of Bone Turnover and Calcium Metabolism in Adults." *The Journal of Nutrition* 133, no. 10 (October 2003): 3130–6. doi: 10.1093/jn/133.10.3130.

National Heart, Lung and Blood Institute. "DASH Eating Plan." Accessed January 29, 2020. NHLBI.NIH.gov/health-topics/dash-eating-plan.

Onvani, S. et al. "Dietary Approach to Stop Hypertension (DASH): Diet Components May Be Related to Lower Prevalence of Different Kinds of Cancer: A Review on the Related Documents." *Journal of Research in Medical Sciences* 20, no. 7 (July 2015): 707–13. doi: 10.4103/1735-1995.166233.

Svetkey L. et al. "The DASH Diet, Sodium Intake and Blood Pressure Trial (DASH-Sodium) Rationale and Design." *Journal of the American Dietetic Association* 99, no. 8 (Suppl): S96–S104. doi: 10.1016/s0002-8223(99)00423-x.

Swain, J. et al. "Characteristics of the Diet Patterns Tested in the Optimal Macronutrient Intake Trial to Prevent Heart Disease (OmniHeart): Options for a Heart-Healthy Diet." *Journal of the American Dietetic Association* 108, no. 2 (February 2008): 257–65. doi: 10.1016/j.jada.2007.10.040.

US Department of Agriculture. "ChooseMyPlate." Accessed January 29, 2020. ChooseMyPlate.gov.

U.S. News & World Report. "Best Diets Overall." Accessed January 2, 2020. Health.USNews .com/best-diet/best-diets-overall.

INDEX

ACKNOWLEDGMENTS

From Maria-Paula

My husband, Chris, and daughters, Victoria and Sophia, are my biggest support system. They are used to my ever-changing schedule, they celebrate even the smallest accomplishment, and in new endeavors, they encourage me every step of the way. This book wouldn't be a reality without their love and understanding of late nights, back-to-back grocery store trips, and extra writing time. I'd also like to thank God, my true companion, my strength. Thank you for listening to me and guiding my words. To my mom, Maria-Paula, and my dad, Pedro, for trusting in me and letting me fly away and grow. To my brother, Pete, who I know is smiling from above because he always knew I was capable of more. Through my career, I've encountered many dietitians who have supported me, believed in me, and guided me professionally. Thank you, Margareta Benser, for seeing in me more than I ever could have. Dr. Carol Ireton-Jones, Nina Salhab, Angela Lemond, Gillian White, Meridan Zerner, and April Clark: Thank you for being outstanding colleagues and inspiring me to be the best dietitian I can be.

From Katie

I live close to my mom, Kiki; stepdad, Bart; and sister, Brianne; because I know that they are always around to offer a helping hand, especially with my son, Milo. With work and a constant to-do list, their support is central to getting it all done. Pam, my mother-in-law, spent each Saturday with Milo to give me the time I needed to write this book and test recipes. I'm so grateful. My husband, Sean, embraced the chaos that came with a new project in a very busy household and supported me and my dreams. Professionally, I have been inspired by a strong community of writers and nutrition professionals. A shout-out to Karina Burnett, Tammy Kling, Angie Griffin, and Melissa Joy Dobbins, who inspire me to write, rewrite, and push forward on new ventures. Thanks also to my incredible colleagues Lana Frantzen, Sara Robbins, Susan Allen, Sarah Ryan, and Jenna Allen. As nutrition professionals and friends, I am grateful for the collaboration and inspiration you bring every day supporting our farmers and impacting our communities.

From both of us

Thank you to Anna Pulley, Kate Slate, and the Callisto team. We've so enjoyed every step of this process.

We also want to thank the support system we have in common, our incredible community of dietitians here in Dallas. Thank you, Neva Cochran, Amy Goodson, Caroline Susie, and Sarah Hendren, for bringing all of us together, supporting our careers, and being outstanding professionals.

Finally, this book would not have been possible without Cindy Kleckner. Thank you for being our mentor, giving us great advice, and meeting with us in coffee shops to discuss culinary techniques. We share your appreciation of the DASH diet and are grateful for all the time you spent with us.

ABOUT THE AUTHORS

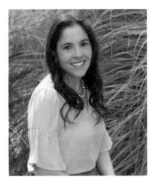

Maria-Paula Carrillo, MS, RDN, LD is a private practice dietitian and the owner of LifeCycle Nutrition in Allen, Texas. Day after day, she focuses on translating the science of nutrition into practical information her patients and clients can use. Having a family of her own, Maria-Paula gets satisfaction from helping individuals and families achieve their nutrition and health goals. She is passionate about her faith, family, friends, food, and fitness.

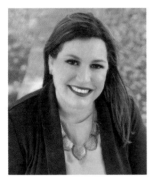

Katie McKee, MCN, RDN, LD is a nutrition communicator working for Dairy MAX. She is a registered dietitian nutritionist and leads a team of dietitians as the director of health and wellness. Katie also has a background in journalism, working as a writer, editor, and reporter before becoming a dietitian. In her work, Katie focuses on simplifying science and empowering people to make small changes that lead to better health. She strives to be clear and concise. She is always working to find a bit of balance in her own life.